LIVING WITH RADIATION

Living with Radiation

THE RISK, THE PROMISE

HENRY N. WAGNER, JR., M.D.
AND LINDA E. KETCHUM

THE JOHNS HOPKINS UNIVERSITY PRESS
BALTIMORE AND LONDON

The Johns Hopkins University Press
701 West 40th Street   Baltimore, Maryland 21211
The Johns Hopkins Press Ltd., London

The paper used in this publication meets the minimum requirements of American
National Standard for Information Sciences—Permanence of Paper for Printed
Library Materials, ANSI Z39.48-1984.

LIBRARY OF CONGRESS CATALOGING-IN-PUBLICATION DATA
Wagner, Henry N., 1927–
  Living with radiation.
  Bibliography: p.
  Includes index.
  1. Ionizing radiation.   2. Nuclear energy.
I. Ketchum, Linda E.   II. Title.
QC795.W24   1989   363.1'79   88-46063
ISBN 0-8018-3787-1 (alk. paper)

We wish to thank Dr. Glenn T. Seaborg for his kindness in writing the Foreword and
Ms. Wendy Harris, Science Editor of the Johns Hopkins University Press, for her advice
and encouragement throughout the writing of this book.

CONTENTS

FOREWORD

The authors present a balanced and illuminating account of the hopes and fears associated with ionizing radiation, extending from nuclear energy and medical radiation to nuclear weapons. They make it clear that a justified fear of nuclear weapons has led to a widespread, unjustified, and unreasoning fear of the beneficial applications of radiation. Although these two aspects of atomic energy are tied together—they both involve the nucleus of the atom and its radioactive rays—a deep misunderstanding of this relationship by the general public has evolved since the time of the atomic bombing of Hiroshima and Nagasaki. The authors' aim is to place the beneficial applications of nuclear radiation in perspective.

Early in the book the groundwork is laid in understandable language of the scientific principles involved, including a historical description of the seminal contributions of the scientific pioneers who made the basic discoveries of radioactivity and nuclear science. This aids the reader in understanding the discussion of nuclear radiation, whose role in our lives is so pervasive but at the same time so generally misunderstood and so unreasonably feared. The inability to understand the value of a risk-benefit analysis leads to a failure to take sufficient advantage of the beneficial applications of radioactive tracers and other forms of radiation.

A strong plea is made for the application by the general public of the scientific method, for which the authors make the case as follows: "Reality is a process of continuous change and bewildering complexity. Resisting change may bring about contentment in the short run, but we risk losing touch with reality. Ignorance may be bliss, but it can also be dangerous. . . . Though far from perfect, the scientific method is an antidote to ignorance, fear, and aggression."

The need for a better understanding of the issues surrounding nuclear radiation is but one aspect of a more general problem. It is fundamental to the effectiveness of our democratic system that our citizens be able to make informed judgments on the more and more complex issues of scientific and technological policy. There can be no doubt that scientific literacy, a solid understanding of science and mathematics, is now more important than ever before. To underscore such a need, the authors cite the still-apt dictum of Thomas Jefferson: "I know no safe depository of the ultimate powers of society but the people themselves; and if we think them not enlightened enough to exercise their control with a wholesome discretion, the remedy is not to take it from them but to inform their discretion."

The authors do not neglect the legitimate "fear" side of the atom. They include an excellent, succinct account of the development of the atomic bomb and the attempts toward its control by international agreements. However, the main emphasis is on the peaceful uses of nuclear radiation, including nuclear power and the many other beneficial uses that are largely unrelated to nuclear weapons—a point that is not generally understood.

The authors introduce an original and intriguing thought that, in a way, relates the two disparate applications of nuclear radiation:

> One of the greatest paradoxes of all time is that nuclear radiation is likely to be our salvation. Radioactive tracers may be what it takes to increase our understanding of the emotions of fear, violence, and destructiveness to the point that we can diminish the dangers of nuclear war. PET (positron emission tomography) studies of the human brain can help us understand better the chemistry of fear, aggression, and violence, so that we can direct our energies in safe and constructive directions toward further human progress rather than a nuclear holocaust. The solution to the dangers of the atomic nucleus may lie in the exploration of the chemistry of human emotions, the chemistry of fear, paranoia, and aggression.
>
> Many people underestimate the risks and dangers of nuclear war, and overestimate the risks of the peaceful uses of atomic energy. They seek to block the development of all applications of nuclear radiation, including the peaceful uses of atomic

energy. They do not accept the premise that radiation can be adequately controlled and used safely for the benefit of the human species. They do not distinguish sufficiently between the benefits of its peaceful uses and the destructive effects of its military uses.

This proposition captures much of the essence of the book. Let us hope that it is not overly optimistic.

GLENN T. SEABORG, PH.D.

PROLOGUE:
THE POLITICS OF FEAR

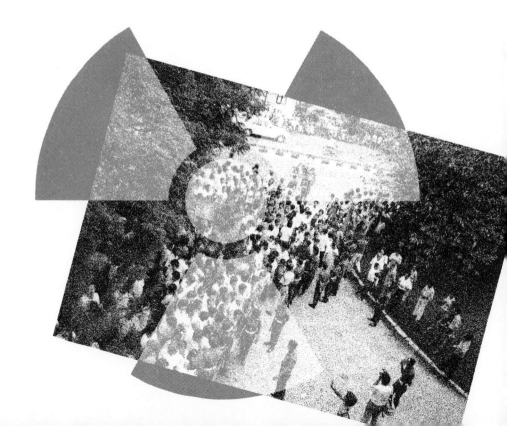

When . . . [people] unite in . . . common fear of one idea, we know it has come to hold deep and secret meanings for each of them, as different as are the people themselves. We know it has woven itself around fantasies at levels difficult for the mind to touch, until it is a part of each man's internal defense system, embedded like steel in his psychic fortifications.

Lillian Smith, 1961

According to cosmologist Edward Harrison, the first law of knowledge is the conservation of ignorance. The more we know, the more we realize how much we don't know. Learned ignorance (awareness of ignorance) takes the place of unlearned ignorance (unawareness of ignorance), but the total amount of ignorance remains unchanged. Cognition and emotion can't be separated, however, and thus ignorance breeds uncertainty, uncertainty breeds anxiety, anxiety breeds fear, and fear often leads to aggression and violence.

The greatest fear of our time is nuclear annihilation. In the words of the late Arthur Koestler, we live with "a kind of psychoactive fallout . . . products of a mental radiation sickness . . . in a world that refuses to face facts. . . . Our species carries a time-bomb fastened round its neck. We shall have to listen to the sound of its ticking now louder, now softer, now louder again, for decades and centuries to come, until it either blows up or we succeed in defusing it."

To most people, the word *radiation* conjures up the specter of nuclear war, a poisoned environment, cancer, birth defects, genetic mutations, even the destruction of the human race. Many believe that radiation and radioactive material can never be handled safely. They will not feel secure until all technology that involves radiation has been stopped. They know that radiation is everywhere, and that exposure to a certain amount of natural background radiation is inevitable, but they believe that anything above natural levels is dangerous. Others find radiation and nuclear technology so complex and seemingly out of public control that they become apathetic or fatalistic. They believe that human beings, like dinosaurs, are doomed to extinction. Their answer to the question posed forty years ago by the English philosopher Bertrand Russell—"Is it possible for a scientific society to continue to exist, or must such a society inevitably bring itself to destruction?"—is negative.

Geologist Walter Alvarez, his father, Nobel laureate Louis Alvarez, and their colleagues postulated that dinosaurs became extinct as a result of profound atmospheric disturbances that occurred when a colossal meteor crashed into the earth millions of years ago. The ensuing explosion was ten thousand times stronger than the potential force of the fifty thousand nuclear weapons now stockpiled on earth. Hot nitric acid poured down from the sky. Falling debris blocked out the sun and brought about the extinction of half of all the animal species on earth at the time, including all the dinosaurs. The disappearance of these species led to the proliferation of the land mammals the dinosaurs had kept "under foot" for millions of years. The previously suppressed species then began to occupy the empty niches left by the destroyed species.

Nuclear weapons, though less powerful than the explosion that wiped out the dinosaurs, could still plunge the earth into a similar sunless ice age. Life as we know it would cease to exist. The earth would be blanketed with smoke and soot, and radioactive dust particles would block out the sun's energy. As astronomer Carl Sagan wrote in 1983, "Cold, dark, radioactivity, pyrotoxins, and ultraviolet light following a nuclear war—including some scenarios involving only a small fraction of the world's strategic arsenals—would imperil every survivor on the planet. There is a real danger of the extinction of humanity."

Paradoxically, the solution to the threat of a nuclear holocaust may lie within the nucleus of the atom. The energy of the atomic nucleus is now being used to explore the chemistry of the human brain and the relationship of that chemistry to human behavior. With new brain-imaging techniques such as positron emission tomography (PET), we can examine not only the chemistry of conscious behavior but also the inner reaches of partially conscious and unconscious behavior. It is not too far-fetched to project that such research may one day provide a better understanding of how human beings think, feel, and act. We may be able to use the new technology to learn enough about the chemistry of fear, violence, and destructiveness to be able to save our species from extinction.

Unfortunately, as we begin to use radiotracers to examine the chemistry of the living human brain and to attempt to understand the effects of that chemistry on human behavior, more and more challenges are being raised to such uses of ionizing radiation. In some quarters, ionizing radiation is beginning to be considered more of a bane than a boon for human existence.

Take the small Malaysian village of Bukit Merah, for instance. What was at first an issue of environmental safety and public health in a small village has become the focus of a decades-old political struggle. The issue is radiation, and scientists and politicians are battling for control.

THE TIN TRIAL IN MALAYSIA

Controversy over the proposed location of a disposal site for low-level radioactive waste near Bukit Merah could result in the closure of the Asian Rare Earth Company's plant that is involved in the extraction of rare earths from the residues of tin mining. The combatants in the struggle include a local Malaysian populace, government officials, and experts from all over the world on both sides of the debate over the nonmilitary use of nuclear energy in society. The outcome of the struggle is likely to affect the process of industrialization in Southeast Asia—and other underdeveloped areas of the world—for many years to come.

Bukit Merah lies in the Kinta Valley of the Malay Peninsula, bordered on the west by the Indian Ocean and on the east by the South China Sea. Flying over the valley from Malaysia's capital, Kuala Lumpur, to the city of Ipoh, one sees vast concentric circles and rows of palm trees, and then acre after acre of jungle interrupted by massive piles of sand. These patterns mark the sites of inactive and active tin mines. Manmade canyons gouge the sandy valley floor, connecting ponds of clear or sandy water to rivers that flow to the Strait of Malacca.

According to Malay legend, a sea captain from Sumatra made his way up the Malay Peninsula via the Kinta River, to the point where it ceases to be navigable. There a genie appeared and crowned him Lord of Kinta, granting him dominion over the world's largest known deposit of tin. Today, that original settlement is the city of Ipoh, and out of a total population of 347,000, 17 percent are native Malays, 70 percent are ethnic Chinese, and 13 percent are Indian minorities.

Throughout its history, Malaysia has gained wealth from one natural resource after another—tin, rubber, palm oil, and petroleum. The world's largest tin mines are found in Malaysia and have, according to historical evidence, been in continuous operation for 1,500 years. During the Bronze Age, tin was used to make drums and axe heads; in the fifth century it was exported to India to be fashioned into religious images; in the nineteenth century it was used by the Dutch to make pewter mugs; and in this century it was shaped into tin cans and automobile parts. By the end of the nineteenth century, 40,000 tons of tin were being extracted from the Kinta Valley per year. The income from tin mining made it possible for the Malaysians to build houses, schools, hospitals, churches, temples, mosques, clubs, and a railway line between Ipoh and the cities of Penang and Kuala Lumpur. During the 1920s, Ipoh had a reputation for "the good life," but by the end of the decade the price of tin had plummeted and an economic depression set in. Today, although industrialization is proceeding at a rapid pace, the country is still not highly developed. Problems of housing, sanitation, and infection persist.

When the Japanese marched down the Kinta Valley on the way to Singapore in 1942, the valley's mines were producing one-third of the world's supply of tin, but Malaysian and British miners flooded the tin mines, putting them out of commission until the Malay Peninsula was liberated in 1945.

The Asian Rare Earth Company (ARE), a joint venture between Malaysians and Japanese, was incorporated in Ipoh on November 23, 1979, and began operating in May 1982, its function being to extract rare earths from monazite sand, a residue of tin mining. The company is owned jointly by a Malaysian mineral company, an organization called Tabung Haji (which finances pilgrimages to Mecca), and a Japanese chemical company, Mitsubishi Chemical Industries Limited (now called Mitsubishi Kasei Corporation). One hundred and seventy-five persons are employed by the plant; both of the plant's managers are Japanese; the rest of the employees are Malaysian. Sixteen different rare earths are extracted from the monazite in their semirefined carbonate and chloride forms and are then shipped to Japan and several other countries, including the United States. After further processing in these countries, purified rare-earth elements are used in making television sets and other electronic devices, computers, and steel.

Most recently, rare earths—particularly yttrium—have been used in the production of superconducting magnets. The 1987 Nobel Prize in physics was awarded to two European physicists who discovered that superconducting magnets can be made to operate at much higher temperatures than has been possible in the past if rare-earth elements such as yttrium or lanthanum are incorporated into the superconducting materials. Some of the new superconductors have been dubbed "1, 2, 3," after the ratios of yttrium, barium, and copper they contain.

Since the discovery decades ago that the electrical resistance of metals such as mercury falls to zero at temperatures approaching absolute zero degrees Kelvin (the total absence of any heat), one of the goals of the world's scientific community has been to discover materials that would superconduct electricity at higher temperatures. The discovery that ceramics containing yttrium and another rare earth, lanthanum, had such properties was a revolutionary breakthrough in physics. No recent scientific discovery has created more excitement.

Up to 1987, access to the practical applications of superconductivity was limited to the privileged few who could afford expensive liquid helium as a coolant to achieve temperatures near absolute zero. The incorporation of rare-earth elements has made it possible to achieve superconductivity above 77° Kelvin, the boiling point of liquid nitrogen—a coolant that is readily available and inexpensive. More recently, scientists in Tsukuba, Japan, at the University of Houston, and at IBM and Du Pont have found that elements such as bismuth can also be used in "warm" ($-243°$ Fahrenheit) superconductors. Subsequently, investigators at the University of Arkansas found that thallium ceramics also were effective, but these results are still preliminary. Nevertheless, room-temperature superconductors are thought to be within the realm of possibility.

Research funds spent on superconducting magnets worldwide total more than $330 million per year, but many technical problems remain to be solved. For example, some of the ceramics are too brittle for most applications. Nevertheless, rudimentary computer circuits and sensors have been built, and one of the many important uses expected of the "warm" superconducting magnets is an enormous increase in the amount of information that can be carried along wires. The information transfer theoretically possible with computers using superconducting materials is illustrated by the estimation that the contents of 1,000 *Encyclopaedia Britannicas* could be transmitted in a single second. Other potential uses of superconducting magnets include trains that travel at great speeds over cushions of magnetism, and improved medical diagnostic imaging devices that operate without ionizing radiation. The latter procedure, called magnetic resonance imaging (MRI), can provide better diagnostic information than existing radiological examinations. MRI is based on a physicochemical process called nuclear magnetic resonance (NMR). (The word *nuclear* was dropped by radiologists because they didn't want a perception of risk associated with ionizing radiation.) Since almost half of all exposure to ionizing radiation is the result of medical X-rays, increased use of MRI should result in a dramatic decrease in the public's exposure to low-level ionizing radiation. Thus it is paradoxical that fear of ionizing radiation may lead to the closure of a plant that extracts materials that could decrease the exposure of patients to ionizing radiation.

THE CASE AGAINST THE ASIAN RARE EARTH COMPANY

The process of mining rare earths is as follows. After tin and other ores have been extracted from sand, the residue, called monazite, contains rare earths and the radioactive element thorium. Monazite itself is not classified or handled as radioactive material, even though thorium comprises 6 percent of its total weight. Prior to being collected for further processing, piles of monazite are found throughout the environs of Ipoh in amang factories. (Amang is the residue of mixed minerals that remains in sand after the extraction of tin.) When the extraction of rare earths is completed, the thorium content of the final residue is 12 percent, twice its original concentration in monazite (6 percent). The final residue is treated as radioactive waste and stored in controlled areas set aside for the storage of low-level radioactive waste. These areas are posted with warning signs and their radiation levels are monitored.

When the Asian Rare Earth (ARE) Company began operating in 1982, the Ministry of Health and Ministry of Industry and Trade

Manufacturing licensed the plant to operate on a trial basis. After two and a half years, villagers from the adjacent village of Bukit Merah obtained an injunction restraining the company from producing, storing, or otherwise keeping toxic and radioactive waste on its land or on adjoining property. With the enactment of the Atomic Energy Act of 1984 by the Malaysian government, and the subsequent formation of the Atomic Energy Licensing Board (AELB) in February 1985, full authority and control over the use of radioactive materials in Malaysia was invested in the AELB.

On November 6, 1985, the AELB formally ordered the ARE plant to shut down until it had applied for and been granted a permanent operating license by the board. The plant remained closed for fourteen months. It restarted operations after building a temporary storage facility for low-level radioactive waste on the grounds of the plant. It also implemented other recommendations made by inspectors from the International Atomic Energy Agency, an affiliate of the United Nations based in Vienna, Austria.

On January 13, 1986, the AELB issued ARE an operating license under the condition that the company construct a permanent storage facility for radioactive waste and have the facility approved by the appropriate government authorities. In the meantime the temporary storage site was to be used. Prior to the construction of the temporary storage facility, the radioactive residues had been stored in steel drums in a trench behind the plant, under conditions that were far from ideal (and that would be the subject of much of the testimony by several plaintiff witnesses in the Tin Trial).

The process of selecting the permanent radioactive waste-storage site precipitated a major political battle, started by the lawsuit brought against ARE by the Bukit Merah citizens' group. Eight residents founded the Anti-Radioactive Waste Committee in July 1984, and began to work with other environmental protection groups: the Environmental Protection Society of Malaysia, the Papan Action Committee, the Consumers Association of Penang, and the Friends of the Earth. Their goal was to shut down the ARE plant.

The ire of the Bukit Merah citizens' group was aroused by the Malaysian government's change in the site selected for the permanent radioactive-waste-disposal facility from an area near a predominantly native Malay population to a region called Papan, located about five miles from Bukit Merah and near a predominantly

ethnic Chinese population. The political implications of the proposed change set the Kinta Valley ablaze with controversy. The citizens' group not only protested the selection of the Papan site but
also charged that thorium waste from the plant had been dumped
illegally in unused tin mine pools and on vegetable farms. The operators of the plant were charged with "exposing the plaintiffs, their
property, livestock and vegetation to serious damage and injury including in the long term cancer, leukemia, genetic injury and
death." The case was brought before the High Court of Ipoh to determine whether or not the plant would be allowed to continue operations, and whatever the decision, it is likely to be appealed to the
Supreme Court of Malaysia.

On the first day of the trial in mid 1987, more than five hundred
protesters against the ARE plant marched five miles from Bukit
Merah to the white-colonnaded High Court building in Ipoh, joining about fifteen hundred others on the lawn of the courthouse and
in the surrounding streets. The protesters, many of them women
and children, marched in twos and fours to avoid being arrested for
illegal assembly. Police vans were stationed near the courthouse,
and about seventy armed police stood guard at the gates and on the
balconies of the building. The demonstrators on the courthouse
lawn cheered as the lawyers representing the villagers arrived by
car at the front steps of the courthouse, and then they booed the
arrival of lawyers representing the company. Throughout the five
court sessions in the first year of the trial (each lasting from one to
two weeks), the demonstrators picnicked on the courthouse lawn,
many wearing white T-shirts imprinted with the words "Perak
Anti-Radioactive Action Committee" written in both Chinese char-
acters and English letters.

The first witness for the plaintiffs described how he and his
grandchildren had been accustomed to taking evening walks
around a pond in back of the ARE plant and had often seen waste
material in steel drums being dumped into the water.

The next witness, a Chinese Malaysian who owns and operates
a sawmill next to the plant, testified that he became concerned
about radiation hazards when he learned of the decision to move
the radioactive-waste-disposal site to the Papan region. He com-
plained that government authorities who recommended the move

had not consulted the local populace, and seemed to have been un-aware of the strong objections that would be raised. The decision aggravated tensions that had existed between the Chinese and Ma-lay ethnic groups in Malaysia for nearly fifty years.

Following World War II, Malaysia was threatened by intense political struggles, including an attempt by the Communist Party, consisting predominantly of mainland Chinese, to take control of the government. The Communist effort was thwarted by the re-turning British armed forces, but the struggle continued until 1969, when political unrest resulted in ethnic riots in which many persons were killed. In the 1950s, "new villages"—including the village of Bukit Merah—were established by the British to separate Malay-sian Chinese from the insurgents, who were primarily from remote rural areas. At that time also, the majority political party in Malay-sia, the United Malaysian National Organization (UMNO), was founded. Its membership is restricted to Islamic native Malays, al-though this stipulation remains a point of contention. Other major political parties are the Malaysian Chinese Association (MCA) and the Malaysian Indian Congress (MIC). Racial harmony has been maintained through an uneasy power-sharing arrangement, the Barison Nasional, a combined front of nine political parties that has ruled the country. Under this arrangement, the Chinese and In-dian minorities have accepted certain restrictions in exchange for being permitted to preserve their cultures and civil rights. Examples of these restrictions include quotas on the number of Chinese who can be employed in certain government companies or can be en-rolled in the national university, and limitations on the use of lan-guages other than native Malaysian in certain public schools.

Recently, the equilibrium among the various political parties be-came strained because of disagreements within the UNMO and a growing challenge to the government from opposition parties, in-cluding the Democratic Action Party (DAP). Attempting to gain strength in Parliament, this party focused on the issue of the safety of the ARE plant near Bukit Merah, and especially on the shifting of the proposed permanent radioactive-waste-disposal site to Papan. The safety of the environment became an important political issue, providing the opportunity for attacks against the majority political establishment. Political leaders, including members of Parliament, joined forces with villagers and environmental groups and invited scientific and medical experts from Canada, Japan, and the United States to participate in a legal effort to close the ARE plant.

RADIATION SCIENCE ON TRIAL

At the beginning of the trial, lawyers representing ARE suggested to the Court that the villagers of Bukit Merah might be "pawns in an international antiradiation battle," a confrontation between those who believe in technological progress and certain environmentalists who believe that most technological development has become a menace to the well-being of the human race, leading to unemployment, exploitation of Third World peoples and resources, the plague of nuclear armaments, environmental chaos, and soaring cancer rates. The international scope of the battle was indicated by the fact that several other organizations joined the Perak Anti-Radioactive Action Committee in seeking to close the ARE plant, among them the Canadian International Institute of Concern for Public Health, the Health and Energy Institute of Washington, D.C., the Japan Congress against A and H Bombs, and the Center for Industrial Safety and Environmental Concerns of India. The last group is a party to a similar dispute involving a rare-earth plant in Kerala, India.

One of the expert witnesses for the plaintiffs was Dr. Rosalie Bertell, who holds a Ph.D. in mathematics and is president of the Canada-based International Institute of Concern for Public Health. A mathematician trained in the United States, but now living in Canada, Dr. Bertell has participated in numerous antinuclear demonstrations and trials involving radiation issues all over the world, and is currently involved in radiation issues related to the operation of a rare-earth plant in Kerala, India. She acknowledges her reputation as an "antinuclear activist," but describes herself as being concerned primarily with public health.

Dr. Bertell arranged for a native Malaysian physician, Dr. Jayabalan, to measure the lead content in the blood of sixty children living in Bukit Merah, the goal of the study being to determine whether thorium was being released from the ARE plant. Dr. Bertell's theory was that since both thorium and lead compounds are waste products of the plant, finding lead in the blood of the children of the village would indicate that thorium was escaping from the plant as well. In fact, eight of the sixty children tested had elevated serum lead values. Dr. Jayabalan presented this finding as evidence that thorium was escaping from the plant and contaminating the children of Bukit Merah.

Testifying a second time, Dr. Jayabalan reported the results of another study, in which the blood lead levels of forty-four children averaged 27.5 micrograms per hundred milliliters (a level that Dr. Bertell claimed was toxic). The plaintiffs argued that these elevated blood lead levels resulted from the children's ingestion of vegetables grown in areas contaminated by lead escaping from the ARE plant. In cross-examination, the defense lawyers criticized the Bertell-Jayabalan study on the grounds that no control studies had been performed on children in other parts of Malaysia, and that lead was not a suitable indicator of thorium contamination. The defense suggested that the elevated blood lead levels could have resulted from air pollution caused by automobiles using leaded gasoline, or from the ingestion of lead paint.

Dr. Jayabalan also testified that he had interviewed forty-three women from Bukit Merah, and that fifteen of the women had lost a child due to miscarriage or perinatal death, both of which he attributed to exposure to radiation from the ARE plant. When his testimony was reported in the newspapers the following day, 1,400 demonstrators appeared at the fence of the courthouse, holding up the newspapers. He further testified that the sixty children of Bukit Merah from whom he obtained blood samples had low monocyte counts in their blood, which he claimed were the result of exposure to radiation from the ARE plant. The defense attributed this finding to parasite infections that Drs. Bertell and Jayabalan had stated were found in the children. Dr. Jayabalan also reported finding that 36 percent of the children he examined had symptoms suggestive of an allergic reaction, and again he attributed this to an immunological abnormality induced by radiation. The plaintiffs ascribed all of Dr. Jayabalan's findings in the village children to radiation escaping from the plant. In cross-examination, the defense counsel attributed them to infections and poor nutrition.

In her testimony, Dr. Bertell cited the results of radon measurements that had been made at the periphery of the plant by Dr. Bernie Lau, a Canadian physician involved in environmental issues.

Dr. Lau's principal professional activity is trying to raise public awareness of the dangers posed by environmental pollution. In Bukit Merah he placed ten "track-etch" radiation detectors near the ARE plant and left them there for four weeks. The levels of radiation he found in the detectors closest to the plant varied between 0.7 and 2.5 picocuries per liter of air, levels that Dr. Bertell stated were evidence of release of radon from the plant.

A third expert witness for the plaintiffs was Professor Edward P. Radford, a retired faculty member of the School of Public Health of the University of Pittsburgh. Professor Radford is well known for his decades-long interest in the biological effects of low-level environmental radiation. During his visit to Ipoh in 1984, Professor Radford viewed the ARE plant from the outside, but never entered the plant or took any measurements of environmental radiation levels. He testified that the plant did not produce radioactivity, but that the process of concentrating radioactive thorium, from a level of 6 percent in monazite sand to 12 percent in the final residue, released harmful radiation into surrounding areas, presenting a hazard to the public. He concurred with the defense's proposition that removing the large piles of monazite from the Kinta Valley, concentrating the thorium by a factor of two, and storing the residues under controlled conditions for storage of low-level radioactive waste would decrease the radiation exposure of the general public throughout the valley.

In his testimony, Professor Radford's principal theme was that the levels of radiation exposure accepted by organizations such as the International Commission on Radiological Protection (ICRP) and the National Council on Radiation Protection and Measurements (NCRP) in the United States as permissible for both radiation workers and the general public are far too high. He stated that his main concern was that the ARE plant was not being operated safely—at least not at the time of his visit—and that the standards for acceptable radiation levels set by worldwide regulatory agencies, including Malaysia's, were too high.

Professor Radford also reiterated his belief that harmful radiation effects in human beings have been detected down to an absorbed whole-body radiation dosage of 3 rems (3,000 millirems). He noted, however, that the observed findings were not statistically significant at radiation doses below 16 rems. (A *mrem*, which stands for *millirem*, is a unit used to measure the amount of radiation energy absorbed by matter, including that absorbed by the human body. One *millirem* is one-thousandth of one *rem*. A *rem* is equal to a *rad*, except for certain types of radiation, such as neutrons, which produce greater biological effects. One *rad* is equal to 100 *ergs* of radiation energy absorbed per gram of matter.)

Professor Radford described his continuing support of the so-called linear no-threshold hypothesis—that is, the theory that no level of radiation exposure is without risk and that biological effects at high levels can be used to predict what happens at low levels of exposure—even when such effects cannot be observed. As a former chairman of the U.S. National Academy of Sciences' Committee on the Biological Effects of Ionizing Radiations (BEIR Committee), he summarized that group's 1980 report. He further testified that the Radiation Effects Research Foundation's 1987 reassessment of the radiation doses received by more than 90,000 persons exposed during the atomic bombings at Hiroshima and Nagasaki supported his position that the effects of low-dose radiation in causing cancer are linearly related to the dose without a threshold below which no effects occur.

The survivors of the atomic bombings at Hiroshima and Nagasaki have been regularly examined and closely monitored for more than four decades to determine whether they and their children and grandchildren have developed genetic abnormalities or present an increased incidence of cancer as a result of radiation exposure. An updating of the results in 1987 indicated that as the survivors became older, the number of excess cancer deaths increased from 100 to 286 per 93,000 persons followed. Professor Radford stated that these and other recent findings support his minority (of one) position in the National Academy of Sciences' 1980 report on the biological effects of ionizing radiation that the relationship between radiation dose and carcinogens is linear down to very low levels of radiation exposure. The majority opinion in that same report was that the relationship was not linear but "linear quadratic," which, if proven correct, would mean that the risk of cancer from radiation was less than that predicted by Professor Radford.

As Professor Radford and the other experts testified, much of what is known about the biological effects of radiation in human beings has been based on the Japanese/American cooperative study of the survivors of the two atomic bombings. Professor Radford believes that the new dosimetry data from Hiroshima and Nagasaki indicates that the risk of getting cancer from gamma radiation (the type to which the public is exposed as a result of medical and background radiation) may in adults be twice as great as, or in young children as much as sixteen times greater than, what was previously believed to be the risk. He supported the recommendations of certain European environmental groups and hundreds of scientists who are clamoring for an immediate revision of the International Commission on Radiological Protection's guidelines for worker protection. Their position is that if the average doses of radiation that the atomic bomb survivors received were lower than previously estimated, then the estimates of the risk of cancer will have to be adjusted upward, in an amount corresponding to the amount that the radiation exposure was reduced. If the new dosimetry is correct, the number of cases of cancer observed in excess of the number expected would appear to have been produced by lower doses of radiation than was previously thought to be the case.

Exactly how far upward the assessment of risk of low-level radiation exposure should be adjusted is likely to be debated by scientists, lawyers, and the concerned lay public for many years. Many experts believe that it is highly likely that for adults the estimated risk from background and medical radiation will be increased on the average by a factor of two, while the estimate of the risk for children could be increased by a factor of ten or even sixteen. The new data suggest that the risk of cancer from radiation exposure after the age of fifty is likely to be considered negligible, while as much as half of the total increased risk of cancer from radiation may be the result of exposure before the age of seven.

If Professor Radford is correct, what is the risk of developing cancer from exposure to radiation? The current belief of many radiation experts is that exposure to 10,000 rems of whole-body radiation increases the risk of dying of cancer by one case. Professor Radford's estimates would at least double this number, and if certain other assumptions are made, the figure could be even higher.

The National Academy of Sciences will soon release a revised report on the biological effects of ionizing radiation. In any case, it is likely that the estimate of the number of deaths from cancer caused by background and medical radiation will be increased over the currently accepted values of 1–2 percent of the total number of cancer deaths.

At the trial, Dr. Bertell testified that Friends of the Earth and hundreds of scientists had petitioned the International Commission on Radiological Protection (ICRP), which recommends protection standards for radiation workers and the general public, to reduce its permissible levels of exposure for radiation workers by a factor of five—that is, from 5 rems to 1 rem per year. Others pointed out that the commission has deferred making any decision for the present, while it awaits the reports of other groups addressing the problem. For example, the National Radiation Protection Board in the United Kingdom is considering decreasing permissible doses for radiation workers from 5 to 1.5 rems per year, and establishing a limit of 50 millirems for the general public.

What would be the effect of such actions? A reduction in the permissible levels of radiation exposure for radiation workers and for the general public would probably not affect greatly the existing industrial uses of radiation, because most worker exposures are already kept well below one rem per year, but further reductions in permissible levels are likely to exacerbate the public's already exaggerated perception of the risk of ionizing radiation. There is considerable evidence that the general public is more concerned about radiation than about almost any other risky activity, including the risks related to cigarette smoking and handguns. If scientists conclude that their past judgments were in error, further doubts will be cast on whether the standards have been lowered sufficiently to ensure safety. The general public would then perceive the risk from low-level radiation to be even greater.

In the past, the genetic effects of low-level radiation were considered by scientists to be the principal concern. Today the principal concern is cancer. In 1956, in an effort to limit the genetic effects of radiation, a committee of the U.S. National Academy of Sciences recommended that manufactured radiation be limited to a level at which the average individual exposure would be less than 10 rems over the reproductive years. The shift in emphasis from genetic effects to risk of cancer resulted from the fact that studies of two generations of children of atomic bomb survivors had failed to find an increase in genetic abnormalities as a result of the radiation exposure.

At the trial, Professor Radford testified that although no statistically significant increases in genetic effects have been observed in these descendants, there is evidence to suggest an increase in intrauterine deaths (presumably as a result of radiation).

In the final point of his testimony, Professor Radford deplored the startup of the ARE plant before the permanent storage site had been completed. He testified that he was not aware that a permanent site for storage of low-level radioactive waste had been constructed in a mountainous region seven kilometers from the plant. A building on the site will eventually house 200,000 fifty-five-gallon storage drums containing the thorium waste. Operating at full capacity, the plant produces about 10,000 drums of waste per year.

Another witness for the Bukit Merah plaintiffs was Professor Sadao Ichikawa, a radiation geneticist at Saitama University in Japan who testified that the measurements he had taken at the periphery of the plant's temporary radioactive-waste-storage site (continually referred to by the plaintiffs as the "dump site") in 1984 had revealed radiation levels that were seven to forty-eight times higher than the 100 millirems per year permissible according to the standards set by the International Commission on Radiological Protection for exposure of the general public. He further testified that the measured levels of radiation at the border of the village of Bukit Merah were two to three times higher than acceptable, and at a sawmill adjacent to the ARE plant were two to five times higher.

Although he stated that he had never been inside the plant or carried out any measurements of radon released from the plant, Professor Ichikawa testified that it was likely that radon was being emitted from the plant. He stated that he did not know why the Malaysian Atomic Energy Licensing Board had renewed ARE's license to continue operating the plant if the factory was not being run safely, or if the board's monthly radiation monitoring had shown harmful levels. He testified that it was almost impossible to prevent the leakage of radioactive radon and thoron gases from the plant and that, in his opinion, the license should not have been given.

Data presented by expert witnesses testifying for the defense and measurements by the ARE Company indicated that there were no radiation levels above background outside the plant. It was suggested that Professor Ichikawa's testimony was politically motivated, as evidenced by the fact that he was accompanied by newspaper reporters and a member of a Japanese antinuclear organization when he conducted his measurements of radiation levels around the ARE plant. Counsel questioned his purpose in bringing reporters to the scene in December 1984 and October 1986, prior to taking his measurements. He insisted that they had followed him on their own. The defense questioned whether it was normal for scientists to have reporters following them when they carried out their experiments, and contended that Professor Ichikawa had turned from science to politics.

Responding to this charge, Professor Ichikawa testified that at the time he obtained his Ph.D. degree in agricultural science, majoring in radiation genetics, he had viewed nuclear power as a promising source of energy. He had changed his mind, however, during his research at the Brookhaven National Laboratory in the United States between 1965 and 1967, when he discovered that small amounts of radiation could induce adverse genetic effects in plants. He testified that when he returned to Japan after his studies in the United States, his findings on the danger of low-level radiation met with opposition and suppression. Funds for further research were no longer made available, he said, because "Japan was then heading towards construction of nuclear reactors and power stations. Many countries including Japan, the United States, and European countries have not told people the truth about nuclear power or made the information easily available to people. The nuclear industries which have all the information should not withhold it from the people in democratic countries."

Professor Ichikawa's measurements of radiation around the ARE plant were performed over a three-day period with a portable gamma radiation dose-rate meter and thermoluminescent detectors placed at twenty-five different locations around the plant. A controversial point in the trial was whether Professor Ichikawa had illegally entered the grounds of the plant to take readings over some storage drums. While a previous witness for the plaintiffs had testified that he had observed Professor Ichikawa making such readings within the grounds of the plant, Professor Ichikawa denied that he had done so, and stated that he had given his dose-rate meter to an environmentalist from the Malaysian city of Penang who accompanied him.

In further testimony, Professor Ichikawa noted that by the time of his second visit to Bukit Merah, in 1986, the plant's temporary waste-storage building had been constructed. Although the observed radiation levels had been cut in half, the storage site was still dangerous, he said. Professor Ichikawa agreed that the thickness of the walls of the building would block any emission of radiation, but he claimed that rainwater was running through the building and carrying radioactivity to the environment. This last point was challenged, however, when he admitted that he had never seen the inside of the building and could not explain how rainwater had gotten into the building.

At the end of the cross-examination, the defense counsel recommended that the judge reject Professor Ichikawa's expert testimony on the grounds that: (1) his testimony that he had not entered the grounds of the plant illegally had been contradicted by another witness for the plaintiffs; (2) he had failed to state that two of his radiation detectors had fallen to the ground (where the radiation levels would be higher) for a period of twelve hours during the time of his measurements; and (3) he had brought newspaper reporters to the site even before he made any measurements, indicating his bias.

Evidence for the defense was then obtained from the manager of the plant and from a radiation expert from Japan, Professor R. Kurosawa, a physicist from Waseda University in Tokyo. Both described the procedures used to protect the workers during the milling of the monazite sand, as well as the results of extensive radiation measurements in and around the plant and over the entire region up to a radius of fifteen kilometers. There was no evidence that radiation levels were above background. During a visit to the plant by experts from the International Atomic Energy Agency (IAEA) at the invitation of the Malaysian government in September 1984, the IAEA inspectors had concluded that there was a "relatively low level of radiation risk involved in this project" but made specific recommendations with respect to the operation of the plant and the design of the permanent radioactive-waste-storage facility. The inspectors approved the start-up of the plant once ARE had complied with their recommendations. They also recommended that "an effective process of public consultation be established, to ensure that the public is well informed, in advance of any proposed (permanent storage) facilities to be approved." After complying with the agency's recommendations and undergoing an inspection of the plant by the Atomic Energy Licensing Board, ARE restarted the plant in February 1986, and it has been in operation ever since.

Testimony was given by the plant manager describing the environmental-control systems used to protect against the hazardous release of radioactive gases and particulates. The milling of the monazite is carried out in a closed system under negative pressure, and thus, the monitored concentrations of alpha-emitting radioactive particles in the air released from the plant can be held at the same level as the natural background radiation measured in the region. Because of the use of multiple filter barriers, the concentrations of alpha-emitting radiation in the water discharged from the plant do not add any radioactivity to the surrounding area. More than ten radioactivity sampling sites within the plant are monitored, and the results are submitted monthly to the Atomic Energy Licensing Board. To date, all have indicated measurements below the permissible levels established by the board's safety regulations. The values have never indicated any threat to public health or safety, and they fall within the regulations of the Malaysian and international agencies concerned with radiation protection.

Monitoring the radiation exposure of workers by means of film badges and personnel dosimeters indicated that the exposure of the ARE plant workers is below one-seventh to one-tenth of the annual permissible limit for radiation workers—that is, the level permitted for the general public (500 mrems per year). The average annual exposure for all workers is 320 mrems per year. Environmental surveys at a total of 295 places throughout the Kinta Valley indicated that the average background radiation level is about 270 millirems per year. The radiation levels in nearby residential areas, including Bukit Merah, were not higher than natural background radiation. No unusually high areas of radiation have been detected around the plant.

Professor Kurosawa provided independent measurements of radon and other environmental radiation in and around the ARE plant since December 1985. The accumulated data demonstrate that "the operation of the ARE plant is safe and protective of the general population and the environment." Another radiation expert providing evidence for the defense was Dr. H. Kakihana, a professor at Sophia University in Japan, and former deputy director general of the International Atomic Energy Agency, who also supported the position that the operation of the plant was safe and protective of its workers, the general public, and the environment.

Summarized, the case made by the defense was that the radiation readings in Bukit Merah failed to reveal any hazard, that the company had been licensed to operate by the Atomic Energy Licensing Board, and that extensive monitoring of radiation levels indicated that the continued operation of the plant and the storage of the radioactive wastes did not threaten the public health and safety. The defense rejected the plaintiffs' claims that milling monazite sand resulted in the production of levels of environmental radiation that were measurably higher than that occurring naturally or that the radiation workers were being exposed to unacceptably high levels of radiation.

The defense emphasized that ARE is a chemical plant and not a nuclear plant, that ARE does not produce radioactivity, but concentrates it by a factor of two times the amount found in the monazite processed to obtain the rare earths, and then stores the final radioactive residues under safe, controlled conditions. The operation of the plant, they contended, in fact decreases the public's exposure to radioactivity by removing all the monazite now lying around the valley under uncontrolled conditions.

The operators of the plant and officials of the Malaysian government emphasized repeatedly that the Malaysian Atomic Energy Licensing Board, established to safeguard the people's health, had approved the continued operation of the plant, that it allowed the plant to operate only under stringent conditions and close supervision, and that it would continue to license the plant only as long as the monthly monitoring indicated that the operation of the plant was not a threat to the public health and safety; if the radiation levels became excessive, the board would immediately close the plant.

SCIENCE AND POLITICS MEET

Whatever its outcome, the trial of ARE in Malaysia is an example of how the fears of ionizing radiation that have become so prevalent in the highly industrialized world are now spreading to the developing world as well, and of how political and social issues complicate issues of public health and safety.

In October 1987, soon after the first sessions of the trial, the Malaysian government, fearing a breakdown in law and order, arrested 106 persons, including the leader of the major opposition political party and several other political figures. Most of those detained under the Internal Security Act were ethnic Chinese, who make up 32 percent of Malaysia's population of 16 million. The Chinese have charged repeatedly in the past that their rights are being eroded by indigenous ethnic Malays, who make up 48 percent of the population and control the country's politics. Among the detainees were the vice-president of the Environmental Protection Society of Malaysia, who was to appear as a witness for the plaintiffs in the ARE trial, and the legal adviser to the Consumer Association of Penang, who is one of four lawyers representing the Bukit Merah residents in their suit against ARE. The session of the trial scheduled for early November 1987 had to be postponed for two months because of these arrests. The government invoked the Internal Security Act, under which it can detain citizens indefinitely without specific charges or a trial. The government justified this action on the grounds that public discussion of sensitive racial issues and the questioning of political dominance by ethnic Malaysians are threats to the national security. Five leaders of the opposition Democratic Action Party (DAP) were forced to resign from their party posts because a section of the Internal Security Act states that a person under an order of detention is disqualified from holding any post in a registered organization.

During the crackdown, a social reform group, Aliran, accused the government of using state-run television to suggest that the detainees had communist leanings. Aliran, whose president was detained but released in December 1987, said that government television broadcasts had misleadingly tried to link the activities of the communist insurgents in the 1960s with protesting groups in the 1980s.

In justifying his invoking the Internal Security Act, Prime Minister Mahathir described those who would undermine stability "in the pursuit of dubious democratic rights and those who ignore the well-being of the majority" as acting against the interest of their country and democracy. "For these reasons, communists and extremists are not allowed to use democratic processes in order to destroy democracy," he said.

The government banned public rallies and revoked the publishing licenses of three local newspapers, including one owned by the Malaysian Chinese Association, which had been detailing charges of government corruption. Subsequently, this paper—the English-language newspaper *Star*—was allowed to resume publication.

Thirty organizations, including the Environmental Protection Society of Malaysia, pleaded jointly for the release of the people being detained under the Internal Security Act. Amnesty International and other human rights organizations declared that the detained persons are "prisoners of conscience." Malaysia's revered first prime minister, Tunku Abdul Rahman, described the government crackdown on dissidents as an action that put Malaysia "on the road to dictatorship."

In March 1988, the Malaysian government issued an official account of the crackdown. Entitled *Toward Preserving National Security*, the report contended that "political parties, pressure groups, the Communist Party of Malaya and the press, exploited ethnic and religious sensitivities for their own selfish interests." This white paper was not accepted by many of the government's critics, and though the government has ruled out any discussion of the document in Parliament, it is likely that implementing the Internal Security Act will continue to be a major political issue.

The tension in the political situation in Malaysia at the time of the trial was further complicated by the prime minister's removing the president of the Supreme Court from office, and subsequently suspending five more associate justices because they had met in the absence of the newly appointed president of the court. According to the nation's constitution, judges can be removed only by the king on the advice of a tribunal. At risk as a result of these actions is the independence of the judiciary.

RISKS: REAL AND PERCEIVED

The trial of the ARE plant is significant not only to Malaysia but also to all developing countries—and to the rest of the world. As the world becomes more and more industrialized, it becomes increasingly necessary to separate real from the perceived risks to individual well-being. What are the real threats to the villagers of Bukit Merah? Should they not be worrying more about political oppression, loss of civil rights, motor vehicle accidents, infections, malnutrition, unemployment, crime, violence, inflation, and nuclear war than about low-level radioactive waste from plants such as ARE? Does ARE increase or decrease their exposure to low-level radiation? Should the villagers accept or reject the operation of the plant? How should they direct their energies toward decreasing the risks they face?

People disagree about what constitutes a risk, the degree of risk involved, and what can be done about it. Estimations of risk can be based on scientific knowledge, but perception of risk involves much more, including socioeconomic, political, and psychological factors. People ignore some dangers and pay attention to others that are much less risky. People often underestimate the risk of diseases, automobile accidents, and violence. In Ipoh, for example, traffic accidents pose the greatest public health problem, followed by infectious diseases.

Factors that increase a person's perception of risk include the degree of involuntariness of the risky activity and his or her unfamiliarity with it, inability to control it, and feelings of being ignored by figures in positions of authority. When people feel that they are not involved in a decision-making process, they are often unyielding in their opposition—even when presented with what would otherwise be convincing data that the risk is acceptably low. Public participation is often too little and too late. When people can participate in risk-taking decisions, they are far more likely to accept risks. If they have been involved from the beginning, they will often accept the legitimacy of decision, even if they dislike the decision itself.

The historical and technological connection between nuclear weapons and the peaceful uses of nuclear energy complicates the decision-making process and the perception of risks involved in nonmilitary uses of radiation. Many believe that the production of nuclear weapons requires the support of nonmilitary nuclear activities, and that the cessation of such peaceful uses would decrease the dangers of military uses. They believe that the existence of nuclear weapons poses the greatest threat to world peace and security, and that the threat would be far less if all such weapons could be eliminated forever from the face of the earth. Others believe that nuclear weapons have been a deterrent to war.

In any case, most peaceful uses of nuclear energy are here to stay. Radioactive materials play major roles in biomedical and pharmaceutical research. Leading-edge research in physics also depends on nuclear reactors and particle accelerators. Some opponents of nuclear technology oppose even these activities, at times accusing proponents of putting their own livelihoods and careers ahead of public health and safety. Others support peaceful uses of nuclear energy, as long as they themselves don't have to live near a nuclear power plant or have a radioactive-waste-disposal site in their town. Most people accept the risk of using nuclear energy to provide electricity, operate a smoke alarm, detect a broken bone or a tumor, discover a new drug, or examine the chemistry of the human brain. A minority of the population does not.

Money, time, and effort are often spent to create and enforce safeguards that are unnecessarily strict. For example, increasingly expensive sites are being developed for the disposal of low-level radioactive waste from medical institutions, research laboratories, and power plants. Estimates of the expense of storing biomedical and other low-level radioactive wastes in the immediate future are as high as $1,000 per cubic foot of waste material. Such restrictions on the peaceful uses of atomic energy are growing tighter and tighter, and are likely to inhibit future biomedical research, delaying or even preventing them from reaching their full potential.

How have we gotten into such a state? In the late 1940s and 1950s, the U.S. Atomic Energy Commission was zealous in its promotion of the peaceful uses of nuclear energy, but failed to deal adequately with the problem of how to dispose of both high- and low-level radioactive waste. The commission promoted the idea that a new era of history had begun, fueled by electric power that would be "too cheap to meter." For decades, its procrastination—and that of political leaders in the U.S. Congress—in dealing with issues such as radioactive-waste disposal strengthened the antinuclear movement.

The villagers of Bukit Merah view the ARE plant as an example of how unacceptable nuclear perils spread from highly industrialized countries to developing nations. The plant brings back memories of the Japanese invasion of Malaya and the atomic bombings of Hiroshima and Nagasaki, and arouses hostility toward business, government, and established scientific organizations.

Fear of radiation can also be found in a paint factory in Arizona; near the nuclear power plants at Three Mile Island, Pennsylvania, Chernobyl, U.S.S.R., Seabrook, New Hampshire, and Shoreham, New York; downwind from the testing of nuclear weapons in Nevada and Utah; at a proposed site for storage of low-level radioactive waste in North Carolina; around the plant of a radiopharmaceutical manufacturer in St. Louis, Missouri; in radon-contaminated homes in Pennsylvania; and in a grocery store selling irradiated mangoes in Miami, Florida. The time has come to make the public as aware and knowledgeable about rems and rads as they are about miles, meters, pounds, kilograms, and seconds.

1

THE RADIOACTIVE PLANET EARTH

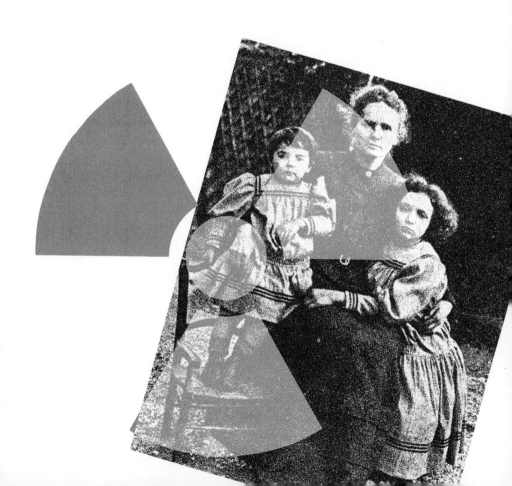

If this thing we call the world
By chance on atoms was begot
Which though in ceaseless motion whirled
Yet weary not
How doth it prove
Thou art so fair and I in love?

John Hall, Epicurean Ode *(seventeenth century)*

URANIUM

The life of each of us is but an instant in the continuously flowing stream of matter and energy in a universe thought to have originated from a single incredibly dense point in space more than ten billion years ago. The "big bang" theory of the origin of the universe is based on observations that all matter and energy in the universe seem to be expanding in a way that suggests that everything in existence began as a "primeval fireball" at one time and place and has never stopped expanding. As one looks back in time at the universe, the density of matter seems to increase without limit.

In 1901, the British physicist Lord Kelvin wrote, "If all the stars through our vast universe commenced shining at the same time [that is, at the time of the big bang] . . . at no one instant would light be reaching the Earth from more than an excessively small proportion of all the stars." The time that it takes for light from the stars to reach the earth greatly exceeds the lifetime of the stars. Therefore, we must be seeing only those stars in the foreground of the universe, not the billions and billions of stars in the distant background.

The star closest to the earth—the sun—is just a tiny speck in the enormous expanse of the universe, which is a vast cauldron of electromagnetic radiation. The light visible to the human eye is a fraction of the spectrum of energy ranging from high-energy gamma rays through X-rays, ultraviolet and visible light, infrared radiation (heat), microwaves, to the longest waves of all, low-energy radio waves. Much of the radiation in the universe exists in the form of "photons," which are discrete packets of energy with wavelike properties. The rest consists of particles. Hans Bethe, a physicist at Cornell University, examined the spectrum of photons coming from the sun, and in 1939 concluded that the sun's energy must come from thermonuclear reactions during which hydrogen atoms are fused into helium. These nuclear-fusion reactions release so much energy that temperatures of tens of millions of degrees are produced. The universe, then, consists of atomic-fusion furnaces burning hydrogen and helium. Carl Sagan wrote, "When we look up at night and view the stars, everything that we see is shining because of nuclear fusion."

Life on earth depends on this continual supply of electromagnetic radiation from the sun. The energy is initially stored in plants through the process of photosynthesis (the conversion of carbon dioxide and water into sugar and larger molecules). Human beings then obtain the energy necessary for life by eating plants or animals that ate plants.

Einstein's famous equation, $E = mc^2$, describes the relationship among matter (m), energy (E), and the speed of light (c). All electromagnetic radiation, including visible light, travels at a constant speed of 186,000 miles (a distance equivalent to traveling seven times around the earth) per second. Einstein deduced from physical data obtained by others that matter contains amounts of energy that are enormous beyond comprehension. The energy from the sun comes from the difference between the mass of the nuclei of four hydrogen atoms, which fuse to form helium, and the mass of the resulting helium nucleus. This difference in mass is converted to enormous amounts of energy, enough to produce temperatures of tens of millions of degrees. At a temperature of 180 million degrees, the electrical forces that normally cause hydrogen atoms to repel each other are overcome, and the fusion reaction becomes self-sustaining.

The conversion of mass into energy is the ultimate source of the energy and matter of the universe. All matter on earth began as the result of fusion reactions in stars. As hydrogen is used up in the fusion to form helium, the temperature of the star falls gradually to a point at which the hydrogen-to-helium fusion process begins to shut down. The helium nuclei can then come closer together, and as they do, more complex nuclear reactions occur, building up elements that have larger and larger atomic nuclei. Helium fuses with helium to form carbon, carbon fuses with helium to become oxygen, and by the successive addition of helium nuclei, neon, magnesium, silicon, sulfur, iron, and other elements are created. The new elements are then swept up into clouds, which later condense to form new stars and planets. Rarer, heavier elements, such as gold and uranium, are produced by intermittent explosions called supernovas.

About three hundred cosmic rays from outer space—electrons, protons, and photons—pass through our bodies every second of our lives. From this cosmic radiation, each of us absorbs on the average about 25 millirems of high-energy radiation each year. The variety of biological species depends in part on mutations produced by cosmic radiation in deoxyribonucleic acid (DNA), the genetic blueprint from which the different forms of life develop.

One of the most momentous events in the history of the human race—equal in importance to discovering the origin of the species— was learning how to convert matter back into energy. This discovery opened two doors: one that could lead to the destruction of all human life on earth, the other to an almost limitless new source of energy. Used as a destructive force, the energy within uranium has become the most dangerous threat to our existence. Used to provide energy and information, the discovery of radioactivity has made it possible for us to explore the greatest remaining mystery of our time—human consciousness. The results of such explorations of the human mind may be the only means by which the human race will be able to avoid a nuclear holocaust.

Albert Einstein once observed that "the unleashed power of the atom has changed everything save our modes of thinking, and we thus drift toward unparalleled catastrophes." Today, we can begin to relate how we think, feel, and act to chemical changes taking place in the brain, and thus begin the greatest adventure of modern times, an adventure that requires the use of radioactivity.

RADIOACTIVITY

In 1669, while searching for the "philosopher's stone" to change baser metals into gold, the alchemist Hennig Brand discovered phosphorus. By the mid 1770s, about twenty other elements had been discovered. By 1800, a rash of new elements, including uranium and thorium, had been found. Uranium possesses qualities beyond the wildest dreams of seventeenth-century alchemists. Few people realize that it is more abundant in the earth's crust than the elements cadmium, bismuth, mercury, silver, or iodine.

Potassium uranyl sulfate, a uranium salt, attracted the interest of physicist Henri Becquerel, a professor at the Museum of Natural History in Paris, because it was fluorescent, emitting visible light after exposure to sunlight. The year was 1895, and physicists throughout the world were excited by the German physicist Wilhelm Conrad Roentgen's discovery of "a new kind of ray," a ray with a penetrating power so great that it could go through the human body and reveal broken bones or foreign objects such as bullets. Within a year of the announcement of Roentgen's discovery, more than one thousand publications about X-rays had appeared.

The rays that Roentgen observed originated at the fluorescent spot where an electron beam struck a metal target. Becquerel had an idea that X-rays and visible fluorescent light might be produced by the same mechanism. He was wrong, but, as often happens in scientific research, the wrong hypothesis led to one of the most important discoveries of all time—the discovery of radioactivity.

Becquerel exposed crystals of potassium uranyl sulfate to sunlight to make them fluoresce. His procedure consisted of exposing a piece of ore to sunlight, laying it on photographic film, and wrapping both in dark paper to record any fluorescence that might have been produced. One day, he happened to develop a film that had been exposed to uranium ore that he had never exposed to sunlight. To his surprise, the film was darkened under the piece of ore even though the sun could not possibly have produced fluorescence. Becquerel's observation, remarkable in its simplicity but momentous in its significance, is a classic example of serendipity, an important discovery made by accident. His simple experiments opened up the new science of radioactivity, and eventually led to an understanding of the internal structure of matter and of the interchangeability of matter and energy.

Becquerel discovered that, like X-rays, the mysterious rays from uranium discharged the electric charge on an instrument called a gold-leaf electroscope. This made it possible to measure the rays, which was essential for further scientific investigation. Like Roentgen's rays, Becquerel's rays were "ionizing radiation"—that is, they were capable of producing ions in air. When Becquerel examined other uranium salts and fluorescent compounds of calcium and zinc with his electroscope, he found that even nonfluorescent uranium compounds produced the rays, while fluorescent copper and zinc did not. The one constant factor in all of his experiments was not fluorescence but uranium itself. Could the element uranium be producing the rays?

Becquerel asked a friend, Henri Moissan, to prepare a disk of pure metallic uranium. He then found that pure metal discharged his gold-leaf electroscope with four times the intensity of the uranium ore. Becquerel had no idea what caused the rays or how they could possibly continue to be emitted even after the uranium had remained in darkness for as long as a year, but he realized the great significance of his discovery. Nevertheless, in 1897 he put aside his uranium investigations and returned to his original preoccupation with fluorescence and optics. It remained for one of the most remarkable women of all time to bring about the nuclear age.

Marya Skłodowska had the characteristics of many creative scientists: dissatisfaction with the status quo, overwhelming curiosity about nature, limitless energy and endurance, and great intelligence. As a teenager, she dreamed that one day she would give up her job caring for the two children of wealthy Polish lawyers and become a scientist. Every day she found time to study physics, anatomy, physiology, and sociology, and one day she received a letter from her older sister, Bronya, inviting her to come to Paris and study at the Sorbonne.

On November 3, 1891, she began classes in the Faculty of Science, registering as "Marie Skłodowska," thus beginning her adaptation to life in France, where she would spend the rest of her days. All of Marie's time and energy were consumed by lectures and study, and after three years she desperately wanted a laboratory in which to carry out her own experiments. A visiting Polish physics professor suggested that she approach the physicist Pierre Curie to try to find a suitable laboratory. Thirty-five-year-old Pierre was attracted by the ascetic young Polish student, and their friendship grew over the next few months. Pierre began to question his resolve never to marry as Marie's intelligence, dedication, and character made him think that love might, after all, be compatible with his life as a scientist. According to their daughter Ève, Pierre vowed to "win the girl, the Pole, and the physicist, three persons who have become indispensable to me." At first, Marie was not enthusiastic about the idea of marrying a Frenchman, leaving her family, and abandoning her beloved Poland, but she finally decided that "we cannot endure the idea of separating," and Marie and Pierre were married on July 26, 1895. Marya Skłodowska became Madame Curie, a woman who was to achieve worldwide fame.

In 1897, searching for a suitable research subject for her doctoral thesis, Marie came across Becquerel's paper describing the new, mysterious rays. What could be causing them? Where could the energy be coming from? The continual emission of energy rays violated all known principles of physics. If she could answer these questions, certainly she would be awarded the sought-after doctoral degree. But what if she couldn't? Should she choose a "safer" subject for her research? Wasn't it too risky to try to solve such a mystery? Her choice of the courageous path rather than the safe and secure one made all the difference.

Marie's first step in the study of the rays of uranium was to learn how to measure them. Instead of using the gold-leaf electroscope, Becquerel's instrument, she turned to an invention by her husband, Pierre, and his brother, Jacques: a new pressure-sensitive crystal that generated electricity when exposed to the uranium rays. With this device, Marie discovered, as had Becquerel, that the intensity of the emitted radiation was proportional to the amount of uranium in the samples. The radiation was not affected by the chemical state of the uranium or by physical factors such as heat or light. To find out whether compounds other than uranium emitted similar rays, Marie examined every element she could get her hands on, and found only one other element that did, thorium.

"We shall call the mysterious rays 'radioactivity,'" she told Pierre, and the substances that produce the rays "radioelements." As she examined one mineral sample after another, Marie observed that the "radioactive" rays released from some samples were stronger than could be accounted for by the amount of uranium or thorium they contained. They seemed to contain a much more powerful radioactive substance than either uranium or thorium. After she had examined all known elements for radioactivity, she became convinced that she must be dealing with a new element, a radioactive element. She told her sister Bronya, "The element is there. I've got to find it. We are sure! The physicists we have spoken to believe we have made an error in experiment and advise us to be careful. But I am convinced that I am not mistaken."

By April 12, 1898, Marie had enough data to announce the probable presence in pitchblende ores of a new element that emitted radiation. Proving its existence was to require superhuman efforts by both Marie and Pierre, who had abandoned his study of crystals to help Marie in her damp little workroom on the Rue Lhomond in Paris. The Curies found that, even in its crude state, pitchblende contained four times more radioactivity than did uranium, yet it was clear that the new element must be present in extremely small quantities, since it could not be detected by the standard chemical analyses. As it turned out, the unknown element made up only one-millionth of the weight of the pitchblende. Its existence was revealed only by the emitted rays. Marie was able to find the new element by chemically separating fractions of pitchblende, measuring the radioactivity of each separated fraction, and retaining those with the highest amounts of radioactivity. Soon they faced another shock: the radioactivity was concentrated in not one but two chemical fractions. By July 1898, Marie and Pierre were sure of the existence of one of the elements. "Could we call it 'polonium' in honor of Poland?" Marie asked Pierre.

In the *Proceedings* of the French Academy for July 1898, the Curies wrote: "We believe the substance we have extracted from pitchblende contains a metal not yet observed, related to bismuth by its analytical properties. If the existence of this new metal is confirmed, we propose to call it polonium, from the name of the original country of one of us."

A second element, which they called "radium," was announced on December 26, 1898. Proving the existence of the two new elements to the satisfaction of the scientific world would require four more years of intensive work. It was necessary to purify huge quantities of pitchblende in order to obtain pure radium and polonium. The extraction process began with ore obtained from the St. Joachimsthal mines, in Bohemia, mines that were later discovered to be the cause of lung cancer in many of the miners. The cost of the ore itself was far beyond Marie and Pierre's means, so they decided to start with the residue that remained at the mine after the initial extraction to purify the pitchblende. Tons of pitchblende residue in sacks were unloaded on the Rue Lhomond, and they began the separation process in an abandoned shed with a leaky skylight across from the little workshop in the School of Physics. "The shed was so untempting, so miserable that nobody thought of refusing them the use of it," wrote Ève Curie.

Marie later wrote: "And yet it was in this miserable old shed that the best and happiest years of our life were spent, entirely consecrated to work. I sometimes passed the whole day stirring a mass ebullition, with an iron rod nearly as big as myself. In the evening I was broken with fatigue."

The Curies' report in 1900 at the Congress for Physics in Paris stimulated great excitement. It was not long before André Debierne, working in a separate laboratory at the Sorbonne but in constant communication with the Curies, discovered a third new radioelement, named "actinium." In 1902 the Curies announced that they had isolated one-tenth of a gram of pure radium and determined its atomic weight to be 225. Radium officially existed; it was spontaneously luminous, glowed with a bluish phosphorescence, and was two million times more radioactive than uranium. The next major discovery was that radium continuously releases a gas, helium. This was the first known example of one element changing into another, a process called transmutation.

Radium defied all the current theories concerning the conservation of energy because it continuously radiated heat. Another discovery was that radioactive elements lose half of their radioactivity over a specific period of time. For each radioelement, it takes a characteristic amount of time for the radioactivity to decrease by one-half, called the "half-life," and for each particular radioactive element, that period of time is always the same. For example, it takes several billion years for the radioactivity of uranium to diminish by one-half. The half-life of radium is 1,600 years. Radon, another product of uranium, has a half-life of four days, and the "descendants" or "daughters" of radon have half-lives in seconds. Without Pierre and Marie Curie, uranium might have remained a simple laboratory curiosity, and the new elements might have remained stored in laboratory collections. The Curies' intense efforts and subsequent discoveries gave birth to the radiation sciences. "Philosophers had to begin their philosophy all over again and physicists their physics," wrote Ève Curie.

The finding that an atom's disintegration is entirely independent of environmental and physical conditions left all prior scientific and philosophical theories hanging in midair. The atom—thought to be the most basic physical structure in the universe—not only was able to collapse spontaneously but also did so at frequent intervals, the process of disintegration being governed only by statistical laws.

Soon it was observed that the newly discovered rays could produce biological effects. Becquerel, carrying a glass tube of radium in his vest pocket, found a nasty burn on his skin under the tube. Pierre Curie exposed his arm to radium and, after a period of time, noticed a change in his skin. Even after fifty-two days the wound had not healed. Pierre's hands began to peel whenever he worked with "very active products." The painful sensitivity of his fingers had not completely disappeared two months later. These biological effects were reported to the scientific world in 1901, and opened up the new field of radiobiology, the study of the effects of ionizing radiation on living organisms.

In 1925 F. L. Hoffman first published his observations of the high incidence of infections of the jaw and marked anemia in women who had been employed in painting watch and clock dials with paint that contained radium and its by-products. These early observations were extended by Martland, Conlon, and Knef, who measured the radioactivity of the body of one of these women, and in 1929 Martland and Humphries reported fifteen deaths due to radium toxicity, including two involving bone tumors.

Despite these reports, a thorium-containing solution called Thorotrast was introduced into medical practice in the United States as an X-ray diagnostic agent used to improve images of the liver and spleen in 1930 (following its introduction in Germany in the late 1920s), accompanied by a warning from the U.S. Food and Drug Administration that its use might be harmful. Its manufacture and distribution were not discontinued until 1976. It has been estimated that between 1928 and 1975 as many as ten million persons were injected with Thorotrast as a diagnostic contrast agent, particularly in the study of the circulation of the brain. Once injected, the solution remains in the body, primarily in the liver and spleen, for the rest of the person's life. Its primary toxicity is to the liver and bone, where it may produce fibrotic scarring of the liver and bone marrow failure. In its 1980 report, the National Academy of Sciences' Committee on the Biological Effects of Ionizing Radiations estimated that 300 excess cases of liver cancer occur per million persons per rad of alpha radiation received. The average dose of Thorotrast gave 25 rads per year. Thus, the risk that liver cancer will develop in a person receiving an injection of Thorotrast is approximately 20 percent. According to Paul Hoffer of Yale University, "Assuming that approximately 10 million persons received Thorotrast, and that 1% received it at a young enough age . . . so that they survived for 25 years after injection [the time it takes for cancer to develop], approximately 10,000 persons have died from Thorotrast-induced liver tumors alone. Yet, when one speaks of radiation disasters, Thorotrast is rarely considered.

Radiation plays such an important part in our lives that it behooves all of us to learn certain basic facts, such as how radiation affects our bodies. When packets of energy called photons are released from radioactive atoms and are absorbed by living matter, energy is deposited in the tissues and cells. When this energy is powerful enough to break chemical bonds, it can cause biological effects. The biological material containing genetic information, deoxyribonucleic acid (DNA), is the most critical target, although chemical changes also occur in the membranes of the cell nucleus. Radiation may affect the cells directly or it may cause changes in water molecules that produce "free radicals," which indirectly damage cells. At certain levels of radiation damage, the cell may die or it may survive long enough to divide once or twice to form new cells but then lose its reproductive capacity. Chromosomes, which contain the genetic material, are a primary site of radiation damage, which can lead to genetic effects or cancer.

What we know about the health effects of ionizing radiation comes not only from animal studies but also from epidemiological studies of populations exposed to high doses of radiation. For example, harmful effects of ionizing radiation have been observed in children treated decades ago with X-rays for *tinea capitis*, a fungus infection of the head, or for supposedly enlarged thymus glands. Years ago, many patients with tuberculosis were fluoroscoped repeatedly in conjunction with lung-collapse therapy; the exposure required high doses of radiation, which increased the risk of breast cancer. Fortunately, such procedures are now no longer carried out.

Other important information about the harmful effects of radiation comes from studies of the survivors of the atomic bombings of Hiroshima and Nagasaki, Japan. Such studies over a period of forty years have led scientists to the conclusion that exposure to one rem of ionizing radiation increases the usual risk of developing fatal cancer—1 in 4—by a factor of 1 in 20,000. If the risk of leukemia is added to that of other cancers, the incremental risk is 1 in 4,000 per person-rem. If all types of cancer are included, the overall risk of cancer from exposure to radiation is twice as great in women as in men. This is due chiefly to sex differences in recorded rates of cancer of the breast, lung, and thyroid. The last, more common in women, is not likely to be fatal. Lung cancer, more common in men, is usually fatal. In the survivors of the atomic bombs, the risk of breast cancer in women exposed to 100 rems or more of radiation was five times greater than the risk in those who received no radiation. In assessing the relative risks of radiation, differences between the Japanese and American populations must be considered. The incidence of breast cancer is very low in Japan; it occurs before the age of forty-five and then decreases, just when the risk of breast cancer in the United States begins to increase. There is a high risk of breast cancer after menopause in the United States, but not in Japan. These differences make it difficult to be certain in assessing the risks of radiation from the study of the survivors of the atomic bombings in Japan.

Since ionizing radiation does not produce a unique type of damage, a cause-and-effect relationship between the amount of radiation received and a given harmful effect cannot be determined by simply examining people who have been exposed to radiation. It is impossible to differentiate the harmful effects of low doses of radiation from the harmful effects produced by other things (for instance, cigarette smoking). In the past, scientists made a significant assumption in order to solve this problem, and many scientists still accept it today—namely, that the harmful effects from high doses of radiation also occur at low doses of radiation, even if such effects have never been observed and cannot be observed. This is known as the no-threshold hypothesis.

If the no-threshold hypothesis is not true for acute lethality, can it be true for cancer? If it were, the same number of radiation-caused cancers would occur among 100,000 people receiving 100 rems as among 100,000,000 people receiving 0.1 rem (100 millirems). This may be true, but it is impossible to test the hypothesis, because so many people develop cancer from other causes. More than one out of every four persons in the United States will die from some form of cancer.

In their efforts to ensure safety in the absence of direct experimental evidence, international and national organizations whose responsibility it is to establish standards of acceptable radiation levels have adopted the "linear dose-effect extrapolation with no threshold" hypothesis. In the case of cancer or genetic effects resulting from ionizing radiation, the safest, most conservative assumption is that there is no threshold. Thus, when one person receiving 200 rems dies of cancer as a result of that radiation, those who have the responsibility of establishing safety standards assume that one of 200 persons, each of whom receives 1 rem, will die of cancer. Although this assumption provides a generous margin of safety for avoiding the possible harmful effects of ionizing radiation, it has also led at times to excessive caution in the use of radiation.

For example, because of fear of radiation, some developing (and developed) countries have chosen to reject nuclear power as a source of electricity when, in fact, nuclear power might have been the best and safest choice. The no-threshold hypothesis can also impede public acceptance of even the minimal risk posed by small amounts of radiation. This hypothesis has led some people to believe that any level of radiation, no matter how small, carries some risk, even if that risk is not measurable. An alternative approach is to assume that a threshold exists unless one can prove with measurements that it does not.

Acceptance of the no-threshold linear hypothesis has created a mindset in the public—and even among many radiation experts—that radiation at the millirem level of exposure is harmful and is a cause for concern, despite the fact that the no-threshold hypothesis has never been proved and cannot be proved. With doses of radiation in the millirem range, as in diagnostic X-rays and nuclear medical procedures, harmful effects, if they occur, are too infrequent to be observed. Therefore, the validity of the linear extrapolation no-threshold hypothesis cannot be tested in human populations. For example, a test of this hypothesis with respect to cancer of the breast would require the study of 100 million women to determine whether an increase in breast cancer occurred following exposure to 1,000 millirems of ionizing radiation. Even if two study populations could be matched very carefully to make sure that those women who received the 1,000 millirems were similar to those who did not, 1 million women would still have to be studied for the remainder of their lives, a practical impossibility. The *New England Journal of Medicine* recently published a report stating that 1 out of 10,000 women develops breast cancer from diagnostic X-rays, but that conclusion was based on extensive mathematical calculations, not on an actual epidemiological study of women who had received X-rays. In view of the fact that 1 out of 11 women in the United States develops breast cancer (from all causes), the increased risk from diagnostic X-rays seems well worth taking.

The increase in the relative risk of cancer from diagnostic X-rays cannot be detected in a given patient, or even in a population of fewer than tens of thousands of persons. Nevertheless, because X-rays may have immeasurable genetic or other effects on the population as a whole, efforts have been made to limit the individual's exposure to them. Diagnostic procedures involving ionizing radiation should be performed only when necessary, but they need never cause fear or uncertainty. Studies in India and Brazil, where levels of natural background radiation are ten times higher than in other parts of the world, have not revealed any increases in deleterious health effects. Such increases have been looked for, but they have not been found. The 1980 report of the National Academy of Sciences' Committee on the Biological Effects of Ionizing Radiations, which examined all the data published up to that time, concluded that it is impossible to determine whether any risk to health is associated with radiation at doses of less than 10,000 millirems (10 rems).

The finding that radiation has the ability to kill living cells and tissues led to its use in cancer treatment. The physicians Bouchard and Balthazard, working with Pierre Curie, found that radiation from radium inhibited the growth of certain forms of cancer in animals. Other physicians then began to try this treatment on humans, calling it "Curietherapy." A radium industry soon developed, and the first factory to produce radium was built in 1904 by a French industrialist. Radium became one of the most expensive substances in the world, its price at that time being $150,000 per gram. All over the world, exploration for radioactive elements was undertaken.

On June 25, 1903, Marie appeared before three examiners of the Faculty of Science of the University of Paris, answered questions about her work, and was awarded the degree of Doctor of Physical Science with honor. That same year, Marie, her husband, and Becquerel were awarded the Nobel Prize in physics.

Although she achieved much success and derived immense gratification from her work and marriage, Marie Curie's life was not devoid of great sorrow. Her husband was suddenly killed in a freak horse-and-buggy accident. Years later, a gossipy newspaper in Paris published love letters exchanged between Marie and a much younger physics student who was married to another woman. The scandal depressed her so much that she considered leaving France and returning to Poland.

For thirty-five years, Marie Curie handled radium and breathed its radioactive daughter product radon. In the spring of 1934 she began to have chills and fever. She grew weaker and weaker, and on July 4, 1934, died of aplastic anemia, a disease of the bone marrow caused by her long-term exposure to radiation. "Her rough hands, calloused, hardened, deeply burned by radium, had lost their familiar nervous movement. They were stretched out on the sheet, stiff and fearfully motionless—those hands which had worked so much," wrote Ève Curie.

THE TRACER PRINCIPLE

Another pioneer of atomic science, Ernest Rutherford, an Englishman, discovered in 1899 that the radiation emitted by uranium consisted of two kinds of rays: one with weak penetrating power, which he called "alpha" rays; and another with stronger penetrating power, which he called "beta" rays. A third kind of ionizing radiation was discovered by the French physicist Paul Villard. It was even more penetrating and, unlike alpha and beta rays, could not be deflected from its path by a magnetic field, which indicated that it did not have an electrical charge. He called this type of radiation "gamma" rays.

Working with the chemist Frederick Soddy, Rutherford elaborated a theory explaining how one element changed into another during the process of radioactive decay. In 1911 he published his concept of the structure of the atom: the positive charge of an atom resided in a tiny nucleus, surrounded by clouds of electrons, a theory that was greatly extended by the Danish physicist Niels Bohr. In the process of radioactive decay, the constituents of the nucleus rearrange themselves, and in so doing eject alpha particles, beta particles, or gamma rays (photons) of very high energy.

One of Rutherford's assignments for Soddy was to separate radium-D from nonradioactive lead. After innumerable unsuccessful attempts, Soddy concluded that the two substances could not be separated because they were, in fact, the same element: "They are chemically identical, and, save only as regards the relatively few physical properties which depend upon atomic mass directly, physically identical also." Soddy coined the term *isotopes* to describe chemically identical elements that occupy the same place in the periodic table of elements. Experiments using the newly discovered isotopes led the Hungarian chemist George Charles de Hevesy to elucidate one of the most important principles in science, the tracer principle, for which he was awarded the Nobel Prize in 1943.

Born in 1885 to a wealthy Jewish family, Hevesy spent his childhood years attending a Catholic monastery school in Budapest. Private tutors gave the eight Hevesy children lessons in German, English, and French, which were spoken on alternate days at the dinner table. School, lessons, and homework took up to twelve hours a day. In those days, children were expected to acquire a large body of knowledge, and had little time left for play, hobbies, or sports.

Hevesy's mother came from the Schossberger family, which owned oil, tobacco, and mining companies. During the late 1890s, the Schossbergers were appointed to a barony. Hevesy's father often participated in hunting parties with the emperor Franz Josef. Hevesy attended universities in Budapest, Berlin, and Freiburg im Breisgau, eventually receiving his doctorate in physical chemistry. He lived a restless life, moving around Europe from one university to another visiting scientists, and returning often to Hungary to spend time with relatives. Because of his family's wealth, he did not have to earn a living, and was therefore able to pursue postgraduate training wherever he found the scientific work interesting.

Historical events—the Hungarian revolution and two world wars—also forced Hevesy to move about Europe. For many years he made his home in Copenhagen and worked with the Danish physicist Niels Bohr, who remained his close friend for almost fifty years. Despite his penchant for working "literally night and day," he found time to fall in love with and marry Pia Riis, a young, attractive Danish woman.

Although Hevesy was financially comfortable, he suffered constantly from frail health. His scientific work was always interrupted by bouts of weakness, whooping cough, insomnia, and depression. He could not live in climates that made him ill, and he spent considerable time in convalescence. When he joined the Austro-Hungarian army in 1915 to fight in World War I, he could not endure his first strenuous march, collapsed, and was taken unconscious to a hospital, where it took weeks for him to recover his strength. Four years earlier, when he crossed the English Channel to work with Rutherford in Manchester, Hevesy had become so seasick that he was bedridden for weeks in London before he was able to begin work in the laboratory.

According to Hevesy, Rutherford "addressed me in his usual unconventional way, telling me that if I were worth my salt I should separate radium-D from all that disturbing lead. Many hundreds of kilograms of lead chloride prepared from pitchblende were stored in the basement of Rutherford's institute. I was then a young man and therefore optimistic. I did not doubt for a moment that I would succeed. When I failed entirely, I had to conclude that radium-D and lead belong to the group of 'practically inseparable substances,' as such substances were called prior to the coining of the word 'isotope.'" What might have remained an impossible research project had been transformed by Hevesy's genius into Nobel Prize–winning work.

Hevesy reasoned that a radioactive substance could be used as an indicator to "trace" the stable element—in a manner analogous to the way a radiotransmitter allows an observer to detect the location and track the flight path of an airplane. In his earliest experiments in 1913, Hevesy used the indicator radium-D to determine the solubility of lead sulfide and lead chromate in water. Radium-D behaves just like lead in water, but its radioactivity can be measured with great sensitivity, and thus it could be used to determine how soluble these salts were in water. No other chemical methods were sufficiently sensitive. Hevesy and Soddy presented their separate experiments employing the tracer principle at the same meeting in England in 1913.

In 1923, Hevesy extended his chemical experiments to biology, using thorium-B, another isotope of lead, to trace the movement of lead from soil into bean plants. The first tracer study in an animal was carried out by feeding radioactive radium-D to rabbits, then tracking the movement of radioactivity through the digestive system to the bones and finally into the urine.

Hevesy carried out all his early experiments using only naturally occurring radioactive tracers. The tracer principle could be extended far beyond Hevesy's most imaginative goals with the discovery of deuterium in 1934 by Harold C. Urey, an American chemist. Deuterium is a nonradioactive isotope of hydrogen with twice its atomic weight. Hevesy obtained deuterium-labeled (heavy) water from Urey and used this tracer to measure how long water remained in the human body. With heavy water, he also measured the rate of exchange of water between a goldfish and its surroundings. Hevesy was the first to propose the important biological principle of the "dynamic state of body constituents." According to this principle, the body maintains its chemical components at a constant level because there is a balance between the rates of formation and the rates of breakdown of chemical substances. He discovered what we take for granted today—that the body is a dynamic and constantly changing, rather than a static, structure.

When he accepted a professorship at the University of Freiburg in 1927, Hevesy fully expected to make Germany a permanent home for his wife and three children. The Black Forest nearby satisfied his need for long walks and nature. He acquired the necessary equipment—including a radiation detector—from his friend Hans Geiger and trained a group of able and conscientious collaborators. Having always felt at home in the society of aristocrats and nobility, Hevesy was not at first alarmed by the political changes taking place in Germany, but he soon realized that Freiburg could not be his home forever and in 1934 he took his family back to Denmark.

The application of the tracer principle took a giant leap forward when Marie and Pierre Curie's daughter Irène, and her husband, Frédéric Joliot, discovered artificial radioactivity in 1934. They observed that irradiating aluminum foil with alpha particles from polonium made the foil radioactive. Their discovery meant that scientists no longer had to depend on naturally occurring radioactive tracers. Artificial radiotracers of practically every element could be produced in cyclotrons (machines that bombard elements with high-energy atomic particles that penetrate the nuclei of the stable elements, making them radioactive) and in nuclear reactors, developed subsequently during World War II.

The American physicist and Nobel laureate Ernest O. Lawrence invented the cyclotron in the 1930s and used it to produce large quantities of radioactive tracers of biological importance, including phosphorus-32 and sodium-24. Hevesy obtained phosphorus-32 from Lawrence to study phosphorus metabolism in rats and human beings, thereby opening up totally new horizons in biomedical research. At that time, the field of radiation safety was still undeveloped, and radioactive phosphorus was sent in ordinary envelopes by regular mail between Lawrence's laboratory in Berkeley, California, and Hevesy's workplace in Europe. Today, such casual handling of radioactive material would be illegal.

The tracer principle, invented by Hevesy, was the seed of "nuclear medicine," the medical specialty concerned with the application of radioactive tracers in biomedical research and the care of patients. Hevesy was "the father of nuclear medicine," and Lawrence, with his cyclotron, was one of the midwives at its birth. Young researchers from many scientific fields and countries were attracted to Lawrence's laboratory in Berkeley because of the opportunities for creative research in biology and medicine that were made possible by cyclotron-produced radioactive tracers. Physiologists and physicians, as well as physicists and chemists, came; among them was Ernest Lawrence's brother, John, who was the first to use radioactive phosphorus-32 to treat patients with leukemia and other diseases of the blood-forming organs. John Lawrence became the "father of therapeutic nuclear medicine."

Glenn T. Seaborg, who discovered many new elements—including technetium-99m and plutonium—and served as chairman of the U.S. Atomic Energy Commission in the 1960s, described the discovery of the medically important radiotracer iodine-131, which is used to treat thyroid disorders:

> In 1938 the late Dr. Joseph G. Hamilton, one of the outstanding nuclear medical pioneers, mentioned to me the limitations on his studies of thyroid metabolism imposed by the short lifetime of the radioactive tracer that was available. He was working with iodine-128, which has a half-life of only 25 min-

utes. When he inquired about the possibility of finding another iodine isotope with a longer half-life, I asked him what value would be best for his work. He replied, "Oh, about a week." Soon after that, Jack Livingood and I synthesized and identified iodine-131, with a half-life, luckily enough, of eight days. . . . It is one of the great satisfactions of my life that iodine-131 has become one of the most useful radioisotopes for the diagnosis and treatment of disease. . . . You can imagine the extent of my gratification when I tell you that my own mother benefited from radioiodine treatment.

2

PLOWSHARES
OR SWORDS?

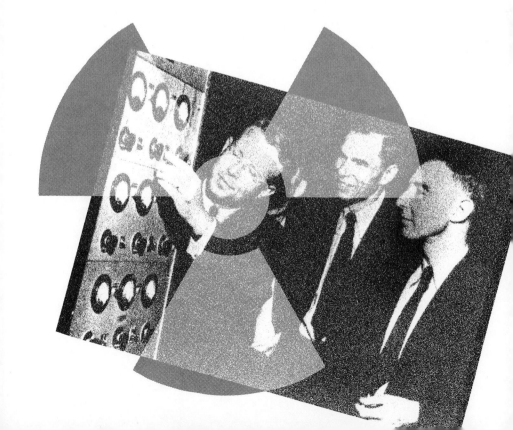

They shall beat their swords into plowshares and their spears into pruning hooks. Nation shall not rise up against nation. Neither shall they learn war any more.

Isaiah 2:4

THE BIRTH OF THE ATOMIC BOMB

The new horizons in biomedical research opened by Ernest Lawrence's invention of the cyclotron in the early 1930s receded as war clouds spread over Europe, but a product of wartime research, the nuclear reactor, eventually assumed the major role as producer of radioactive tracers. In 1939, the famous Danish physicist Niels Bohr arrived in Princeton, New Jersey, bearing the startling news that the German physical chemists Otto Hahn and Fritz Strassman had produced barium, krypton, and other elements by bombarding uranium with neutrons. Neutrons had been discovered by James Chadwick in England seven years earlier, when he bombarded the element beryllium with alpha particles emitted from polonium. Chadwick observed the release of uncharged nuclear particles that had the same mass as positively charged protons. The new particles, which he named "neutrons," eventually made it possible to split the atom and unlock the enormous energy within the atomic nucleus. Even before the discovery of neutrons, scientists had been able to obtain glimpses of the energy within the atom when they bombarded beryllium with charged alpha particles, but the energy consumed in the process was greater than that released. No one had been able to produce a self-sustaining "chain reaction" that would release the energy that they knew lay hidden within the atom, as predicted by Einstein's equation $E = mc^2$. The key lay in the uncharged neutrons, which could enter the highly charged atomic nucleus more readily than could the highly charged alpha particles.

Lise Meitner and Otto Frisch, two of many physicists who fled to Denmark from Germany because of Hitler's persecution of the Jews, provided the scientific world with the explanation of the findings that Hahn and Strassman had reported: "It seems possible that the uranium nucleus . . . may, after neutron capture, divide itself into two nuclei of roughly equal size. . . . These two nuclei . . .

should gain a total kinetic energy of (about) 200 MeV." If more free neutrons were created than were consumed in splitting the atom, a self-sustaining chain reaction might be achieved, and the enormous energy within the nucleus might be released.

At almost the same time, two American scientists, R. D. Fowler and R. W. Dodson, of the Johns Hopkins University, reported in the British journal *Nature* that they had actually observed with an ionization chamber the particles released by the disintegration of uranium. They reported that three or four neutrons were released from each uranium atom that split. All over Europe—in France, England, and Germany—scientists filed patents and made arrangements to obtain uranium from the Belgian Congo, even though most physicists doubted that a chain reaction could actually be achieved. Ernest Lawrence himself said that the prospect of producing energy from the atom was as remote as that of cooling the ocean and putting its heat to work. Rutherford summed up the situation, saying, "The outlook for gaining useful energy by artificial processes of transformation does not look promising." (Admiral William Leahy was to say later that the proposed project to develop an atomic bomb was "the biggest fool thing we have ever done.")

Some atomic scientists became greatly concerned about the possibility that German scientists might be able to develop an atomic bomb. One physicist, the Hungarian Leo Szilard, learned of the revolutionary experiments of Hahn and Strassman and other physicists, and, fearing a nuclear arms race, traveled immediately to the United States and enlisted the aid of the Italian physicist Enrico Fermi. After accepting the 1938 Nobel Prize in physics, Fermi had emigrated directly from Stockholm to the United States to join another immigrant, Isidor Rabi, a physicist at Columbia University whose family had left Galacia for New York in the late 1890s, when he was an infant. After receiving his Ph.D. degree in physics from Columbia University, Rabi had traveled to Europe to be with scientists who were developing the field of quantum mechanics. Upon his return to Columbia in 1929, he began his experimental studies of the atomic nucleus, which eventually culminated in his being awarded the Nobel Prize in physics in 1944.

At first, even Fermi was not convinced that a nuclear chain reaction could be achieved. But Szilard, working in a guest laboratory at Columbia University, proved experimentally that from every uranium atom undergoing fission, at least two neutrons were emitted for every captured neutron. Therefore, a nuclear chain reaction was indeed possible. Fermi's calculations showed that one pound of uranium would be capable of yielding as much energy as three million pounds of coal.

With this evidence in hand, Fermi went to Washington, D.C., to meet with the assistant secretary of the Navy to request funds to try to find out whether a chain reaction could be induced in a *large* mass of uranium. Fermi was unsuccessful in getting the funds, but Szilard persisted because he was obsessed with the idea that nuclear weapons could be made and might fall into the hands of the German government. Even more frightening to him was the news that the Germans had seized control of the uranium mines in Czechoslovakia in the spring of 1939 and had immediately forbidden the export of uranium ore.

Accompanied by his Hungarian colleagues Eugene Wigner and Edward Teller, Szilard drove to see Albert Einstein, who was vacationing on Long Island. After listening to Szilard's evidence that an atomic bomb might be possible, Einstein agreed to write a letter to the Belgian government to warn them of the danger of selling uranium ore to the Germans. First, however, Szilard and Einstein decided that they should get the approval of the U.S. State Department to send the letter. Szilard then sought the help of economist Alexander Sachs, a close friend of President Roosevelt. Immediately grasping the significance of his visitor's concerns, Sachs advised Szilard not to go through the State Department but to ask Einstein to write directly to President Roosevelt. Sachs said that he would be willing to deliver the letter personally.

In his letter to Roosevelt, Einstein wrote:

> Some recent work by E. Fermi and L. Szilard, which has been
> communicated to me in manuscript, leads me to expect that
> the element uranium may be turned into a new and important
> source of energy in the immediate future. Certain aspects of
> the situation seem to call for watchfulness and, if necessary,
> quick action on the part of the administration. . . . It may
> become possible to set up nuclear chain reactions in a large
> mass of uranium, by which vast amounts of power and large

quantities of new radium-like elements will be generated. . . . This new phenomenon could also lead to the construction of bombs. . . . A single bomb of this type, carried by boat or exploded in a port, might very well destroy the whole port together with some of the surrounding territory [he did not imagine the magnitude of the nuclear weapons that would eventually be built].

Einstein suggested that the government immediately help American scientists in universities and industries obtain a supply of uranium ore and begin experimental work on atomic fission. He cited rumors that the Germans were "engaged in secret work involving atomic research directed toward achievement of a nuclear chain reaction." It took two visits to the White House by Sachs on consecutive days to convince Roosevelt that (in Roosevelt's words) "what you are after is to see that the Nazis don't blow us up." The initial experiments cost $6,000 and were designed to see whether a graphite-uranium system could develop a chain reaction.

When Germany invaded Belgium and imperiled the supply of uranium from the Belgian Congo, Sachs went back to see Roosevelt to expedite the program. On June 15, 1940, Roosevelt agreed to put the atomic bomb project under the Office of Scientific Research and Development, headed by Vannevar Bush, a distinguished scientist and president of the Carnegie Institute of Washington. In December 1941, the month of the Japanese attack on Pearl Harbor, President Roosevelt formed a three-person "Uranium Committee," with instructions to go full speed ahead to build the first atomic bomb and to establish a research-and-development program in atomic energy. By August 13, 1942, the Manhattan Engineering District Project had been established in the Army Corps of Engineers, with General Leslie Groves as its chief. Its charge was to develop an atomic bomb as rapidly as possible.

The person chosen by Groves to make the bomb was the physicist J. Robert Oppenheimer, from Ernest Lawrence's laboratory in Berkeley, California. The site Oppenheimer selected for the project was the Los Alamos Ranch School for Boys, in the remote mountains of New Mexico, which he had visited as a child. Oppenheimer recruited the best scientists in the country to work on the project, and his leadership transformed them into an effective team. He described the atmosphere at the laboratory as follows: "Almost every-one knew that this job, if it were achieved, would be part of history. This sense of excitement, of devotion, and of patriotism in the end prevailed."

By late 1942, the American scientists and their refugee col-leagues at Los Alamos and elsewhere were becoming desperate be-cause they had made little progress. Secret reports continued to ar-rive, informing them that large consignments of uranium and heavy water were entering Germany every week, falling into the hands of atomic scientists whom they believed were the best in the world. To progress, the Americans needed pure uranium-235, be-cause a chain reaction could be induced only by bombarding ura-nium with neutrons to split the uranium-235 atoms, thereby releas-ing more neutrons to react with other uranium-235 atoms until a self-sustaining chain reaction occurred. American industry re-sponded to the challenge, and in November 1942, the Westinghouse Corporation delivered three tons of purified uranium to Fermi and his scientific colleagues at a squash court beneath the west stands of Stagg Field, at the University of Chicago. There they began con-struction of the first nuclear "pile."

At 3:30 P.M. on December 2, 1942, Fermi gave the signal for the withdrawal of the last "control" rod of the world's first nuclear reac-tor. The increasing intensity of the clicking of radiation detectors signified that "criticality" had been reached, each successive genera-tion of neutrons exceeding the last in the first man-made nuclear chain reaction in history.

The construction and testing of the first atomic bomb lay ahead. Secrecy had to be maintained at all costs. Most of the scientists and contractors on the project throughout the country had no idea what they were working on. The man most closely watched was Oppenheimer himself. He had close relatives who were members of the Communist Party, and had been engaged to be married to a known Communist who had committed suicide. Oppenheimer's patriotism was often questioned, but there was never any evidence that he was a Communist or accepted Communist beliefs. At one point, General Groves told the Federal Bureau of Investigation, "Young people who attended a Communist meeting or two and later realized their mistakes should not be damned forever."

The concern over Oppenheimer was an example of misplaced efforts to keep atomic secrets from the Soviet Union. The real Communist spy at Los Alamos was Klaus Emil Fuchs, a highly gifted physicist in the inner circle of the top scientists. Fuchs was a native German who had fled to England and become a British citizen. His loyalty to the Allied war effort was never questioned during the war, but after the war he provided Moscow with the information needed to produce an atomic bomb.

The Manhattan District Project involved universities, government, and industry all over the country, and had cost more than two billion dollars by the time the test explosion of the first atomic bomb was carried out in the New Mexico desert on July 16, 1945. At 5:30 A.M. the bomb exploded with an enormous flash of light, vaporizing the tower on which it stood. Thirty seconds later, the observers, safely huddled a mile away, were jarred by a wind of hurricane force, followed by a deafening roar that swept across the desert. One observer, William L. Laurence, described

> a sunrise such as the world had never seen, a great green supersun climbing in a fraction of a second to a height of more than eight thousand feet, rising ever higher until it touched the clouds, lighting up earth and sky all around with a dazzling luminosity. Up it went, a great ball of fire about a mile in diameter, changing colors as it kept shooting upward, from deep purple to orange, expanding, growing bigger, rising as it expanded, an elemental force freed from its bonds after being chained for billions of years. For a fleeting instant the color was an unearthly green, such as one sees only in the corona of the sun during a total eclipse. It was as though the earth had opened and the skies had split. One felt as though one were present at the moment of creation when God said: "Let there be light."

Within a mile of the bomb blast all plant and animal life—including cactuses, desert grass, and rattlesnakes—was destroyed. An antelope herd vanished. Oppenheimer was reminded of a passage from the Bhagavad-Gita: "I am become Death, the shatterer of worlds."

The following message was delivered immediately to Secretary of War Henry Lewis Stimson, who was meeting with leaders of the

Four Powers in Potsdam: "Operated on this morning. Diagnosis not yet complete but results seem satisfactory." Two days later, a second message arrived: "Doctor has just returned most enthusiastic and confident that the little boy is as husky as his big brother."

THE DECISION TO USE THE BOMB

Officials of the U.S. government debated the wisdom of telling the Soviets about the bomb. They finally decided that President Truman should tell Stalin that the United States had a new weapon of unusual destructive force, but that he should not elaborate. Stalin said that he was glad to hear it, and hoped that the Americans would make "good use of it against the Japanese."

Many scientists, including Leo Szilard, strongly opposed the atomic bombing of Japanese cities. They believed it would stigmatize the United States for all time. The Soviet Union, knowing that in a future war Americans might drop atomic bombs on them, could be expected to build atomic weapons of its own at all costs, spurring a disastrous, uncontrollable arms race.

Before the first test of the atomic bomb at Alamogordo, New Mexico, Szilard asked Edward Teller, who was working under Robert Oppenheimer's direction at Los Alamos, to collect the signatures of those scientists who were opposed to using the atomic bomb on the Japanese people without warning. Such a petition had already been signed by many scientists on the Chicago team that had developed the first nuclear reactor. Believing that it was improper for a scientist to use his prestige as a platform for political statements, Teller never circulated the petition. In his autobiography, written seventeen years later, Teller stated that he later regretted not doing so.

Teller and Szilard were both born in Budapest, attended the same high school, emigrated to the United States to escape anti-Semitic fascism in Europe, and worked on the development of the atomic bomb. Despite their common background and activities, however, their personalities were quite different, and they eventually expressed diametrically opposed political viewpoints. An extrovert with a strong social conscience, Szilard became the champion of collaboration between the United States and the Soviet Union in using atomic energy in the search for world peace. Teller was much more of a loner, and eventually became the champion of a hard-line approach to the Soviets in the postwar period. He assumed the major responsibility for developing the hydrogen bomb, which was opposed by Szilard, Oppenheimer, Fermi, Rabi, and other scientists.

Another person who opposed the atomic bombing of Japan was Admiral William Leahy, chairman of the Joint Chiefs of Staff and a personal confidant of President Truman. Leahy believed that dropping the bomb on a Japanese city would increase the likelihood that some day, some enemy might emulate the United States and drop atomic bombs on American cities. The Japanese were about to surrender, having been beaten by the sea blockade and by saturation bombings with conventional weapons. Leahy and other military experts believed that an invasion of the Japanese mainland would be unnecessary because most Japanese war and merchant ships had been sunk and most major cities in Japan lay in ruins. They argued that a tighter sea blockade and more conventional pinpoint bombing would bring about an almost immediate surrender. They believed that Japan would surrender if the Soviet Union did no more than simply declare war. General George Marshall also believed that "playing the Soviet card" would obviate the need for the use of the atomic bomb. He advocated waiting to see whether a Soviet invasion would trigger a Japanese surrender. Evidence obtained from both Japanese and American sources after the war suggests that most military experts thought that an invasion was unnecessary.

Secretary of War Stimson believed that it would be impossible to plan a better "new world" if a hundred thousand human beings were massacred in an instant. He advocated making a direct offer to the Soviet Union to participate in the further development and control of atomic energy, and to subsequently try to bring other nations into the agreement. He believed that unless some progress toward international control was made immediately, a nuclear arms race was inevitable. Stimson then reiterated the argument set forth in a letter sent to President Truman by O. C. Brewster, a scientist who had worked on the bomb: if the United States set a precedent by dropping the first atomic bomb, Americans would become the most hated and feared people on the earth, and some "corrupt and venal demagogue" would one day try to destroy the world with the weapon for his own insane satisfaction.

A committee of scientists chaired by James Franck, including Szilard and Seaborg, supported the position that secrecy and attempts to corner the supply of raw materials to make atomic bombs would be futile, and that the only hope for safety lay in international control. The Franck committee recommended that nuclear weapons not be used against the Japanese without warning, because such a course of action would cost the United States support throughout the world, precipitate a nuclear arms race, and decrease the chances of ever achieving an international agreement on control of nuclear energy and weapons. The committee favored a demonstration of the bomb in some uninhabited area. It advocated developing this "new frontier" with a minimum of secrecy, and in cooperation with other world powers, so that atomic energy might become a force for peace. In its judgment, use of the bomb in combat would ultimately preclude the international control of nuclear weapons.

By the time the Franck report was submitted to the government, President Truman and the executive department had already taken the position that the cost in human lives of invading Japan could be avoided by using the bomb. In their view, demonstrating the bomb's deadly effectiveness would increase, rather than decrease, the likelihood of eventually achieving international control.

One of the people who played a crucial role in the decision to drop atomic bombs on Hiroshima and Nagasaki was President Truman's closest adviser, Secretary of State James Byrnes, who viewed the bomb as the key to postwar Soviet-American relations. Byrnes believed that prior secret agreements between President Roosevelt and Premier Joseph Stalin at Yalta had unfortunately given the Soviet Union the go-ahead to communize Poland and split Europe into two spheres of influence. In the effort to persuade the Soviet Union to declare war on Japan, the Allies had agreed to give the Soviets the eastern end of the Trans-Siberian Railway in Manchuria, the Kurile Islands, half of Sakhalin Island (another island north of Japan), an occupation zone in Korea, veto power at the United Nations, U.N. seats for the Ukraine and Byelorussia, and recognition of the autonomy of Outer Mongolia. Byrnes further believed that the ailing President Roosevelt had been hoodwinked by Stalin at Yalta, and that only by dropping the atomic bomb could the United States turn back the clock. Byrnes predicted that just as Americans had bowed to Soviet power at Yalta, the Soviets would bow to American power after the bombing of Hiroshima and Nagasaki. Atomic bombs exploding over Japan would "teach Stalin how far the Soviets could go," and would guarantee American dominance in the world of the future. The Soviets would be forced to remove their troops from Poland, Hungary, and Rumania, and "might be more manageable if impressed by American military might."

General Groves advised the government that the Soviet Union would be unable to develop an atomic bomb for another twenty years; others had estimated three to five years. Byrnes's position was that if Stalin were given information about the bomb right away, he would ask for full rights as an atomic partner with the United States and Britain. Byrnes believed that "[an] international agreement was not practical and that Oppenheimer and the rest of the gang should pursue their work [on the hydrogen bomb] at full force." In Byrnes's view, the atomic bomb was just another devastating weapon that could be assimilated into international relations.

"I shared Byrnes' concern about Russia's throwing her weight around in the postwar period," Szilard later wrote, "but I was completely flabbergasted by the assumption that rattling the bomb might make Russia more manageable." Indeed, as Szilard had predicted, the bombing of Japan was to precipitate an arms race that has lasted for nearly half a century. Nothing could have made the Soviets move faster to build their own nuclear weapons than the Americans' use of the bomb against Japan.

And so, orders went out to the 509th Composite Group to drop the atomic bomb on one of four Japanese cities—Hiroshima, Kokura, Nugata, and Nagasaki—as soon after August 3, 1945, as weather permitted. The other three cities were to be attacked as soon as bombs became available.

On July 26 the cruiser *Indianapolis* delivered the uranium-235 bomb "Little Boy" to Tinian Island, in the Pacific. The bomb was 28 inches in diameter and 120 inches long, weighed 9,000 pounds, and had an equivalent yield of 20,000 tons of high explosives. Three transport planes flew in other essential components over the next three nights, and on July 31 "Little Boy" was ready.

On August 6, 1945, the first atomic bomb used in warfare was detonated over Hiroshima, Japan, and on August 9, 1945, a second atomic bomb, called "Fat Man"—the last used in warfare—was dropped over Nagasaki. The second bomb was to have been dropped on August 11, but the commanding officer of the 509th Composite Group received permission to advance the schedule by two days to avoid a five-day stretch of bad weather that had been forecast. A third atomic bomb was being prepared for transport from Los Alamos.

On August 8 the Japanese ambassador to the Soviet Union called on Vyacheslav Molotov, the Soviet foreign minister, to plead for Soviet mediation of an agreement with the United States to end the war. Instead, he was told that as of August 9, the Soviet Union would consider itself at war with Japan. That same day Emperor Hirohito and his ministers accepted the terms for surrender, which had previously been set forth by the Americans at Potsdam amid rumors that Tokyo was scheduled for an atomic bombing on August 12. Word was sent to the United States through Switzerland and Sweden that Japan had accepted the Potsdam terms provided the emperor could remain as sovereign ruler. Later that day Japanese government officials in Tokyo learned of the attack on Nagasaki.

At 7:00 P.M. on Tuesday, August 14, the war was over. The atomic bomb had had an immediate effect, but many people believed that America's ability to lead the nations of the world in a cooperative effort to lessen the threat of a nuclear holocaust had been severely impaired.

INTERNATIONAL CONTROL OF ATOMIC ENERGY

Attempts to achieve international control of atomic energy and avoid a nuclear arms race almost succeeded. Newspapers around the world heralded "a new age, the Atomic Age." Atomic energy had moved from the realm of science into full public view. Robert Hutchins, of the University of Chicago, was a staunch advocate of the internationalization of atomic energy, believing that "only through the monopoly of atomic force by world government can we hope to abolish war." On March 28, 1946, Secretary of State Dean Acheson and David Lilienthal, the future chairman of the U.S. Atomic Energy Commission, issued a report supporting international control of all aspects of nuclear energy, including weapons. In general, the response of the general public was favorable, but influential newspapers such as the *Chicago Tribune* and the *Washington Times Herald* denounced the report as a pernicious scheme to give the secrets of the atomic bomb to the Soviets. On the other side, the *Washington Post* viewed the report as offering hope for lifting the "Great Fear" that had descended over the world the previous summer.

On June 14, 1946, Bernard Baruch presented a formal proposal to the United Nations to establish an organization called the International Atomic Energy Commission, which was to be entrusted with all phases of the development and use of atomic energy. The plan was to have France and China join the other permanent members of the U.N. Security Council: the United States, the United Kingdom, and the Soviet Union. The international commission was to make proposals in stages for exchanging basic scientific information, confining atomic energy to peaceful purposes, eliminating atomic and other weapons of mass destruction from national armaments, and safeguarding the states that complied. The commission would exercise managerial control or ownership of all nuclear materials threatening world security. It would have the power to control, inspect, and license all nuclear facilities, foster beneficial uses of atomic energy, and assume responsibility for atomic research and development.

Most nations favored total international control of both peaceful and military uses of nuclear energy, but the Soviets feared that the U.S. proposal for international control was simply a mechanism intended to perpetuate their monopoly of the development of nuclear weapons. They feared that attempts at international control would not only fail but would also inhibit their own development of nuclear weapons. In the Soviets' view, such a state of affairs would be too dangerous in light of the United States' monopoly and obvious willingness to use atomic weapons. The plan to achieve international control of nuclear energy foundered on the specific issue of whether sanctions for violations of the international agreements would be subject to a veto by any member of the U.N. Security Council. Bernard Baruch, representing the United States at the negotiations, supported the position that "there shall be no legal right, by veto or otherwise, whereby a willful violator of the terms of the treaty or convention shall be protected from the consequences of violation of its terms." The representative of the Soviet Union, Andrei Gromyko, charged that the American position of prohibiting the veto violated a basic principle of the Charter of the United Nations.

The opposing American and Soviet positions on the question of veto power in the enforcement of the treaty became a major stumbling block, and this was used as an excuse by the Soviets to reject the entire proposal despite the fact that support for it by the international community was overwhelming. American insistence on abolishing the veto in the case of violations led some people to conclude that the United States was not sincere in its efforts to achieve international control of nuclear energy.

Some of the leading nuclear physicists who had developed the bomb were convinced that the Soviet Union and the other great powers would never permit the United States to continue to monopolize the field of atomic weaponry, with or without the efforts at international control through the United Nations. They believed that the salvation of the human species lay in making sure that no nation could ever again produce fissionable material in a form suitable for weapons. The only way to prevent nuclear war would be to outlaw all nuclear activities, a position that is taken today by many antinuclear activists. Other scientists who had worked on the development of the bomb, including Ernest Lawrence, the inventor of the cyclotron, took the position that nuclear research in the United States should proceed unceasingly—that by strenuous efforts the United States could maintain its lead. Lawrence proposed stockpiling uranium for military and industrial uses and encouraging the development of further industrial uses for nuclear energy. Leo Szilard was a leading spokesman for the opposition, which was convinced that people like Lawrence did not grasp the true significance of atomic weapons. President Truman and Secretary of State James Byrnes took the view that "world cooperation for peace will soon reach such a state of perfection that atomic methods of destruction can be definitely and effectively outlawed forever." Their words suggest that they did not believe the time had yet come to try to develop enforceable international agreements to outlaw nuclear weapons.

The fact that the United States was simultaneously drafting an agreement with England to share information on the production of nuclear weapons reflected poorly on the sincerity of the Americans and British in fostering an international effort to control such weapons. In a joint directive, the United States, the United Kingdom, and Canada pledged "full and effective cooperation in the field of atomic energy."

An event that helped shatter the hopes for international cooperation occurred on February 16, 1946. Twenty-two people were arrested in Canada for leaking "atomic bomb secrets" to the Soviet embassy. The news was taken as further evidence of Russian perfidy, and dealt the previous agreement between the Soviet Union and the United States a serious blow. The news was a psychological shock to both the U.S. Congress and the public. Fear again arose to drown out the postwar idealism that might have led to international control of nuclear weapons. What happened instead set the stage for a nuclear arms race that continues to this day.

When the Soviet Union tested its first atomic bomb in 1949, Edward Teller resumed promoting the development of the hydrogen bomb. His most enthusiastic supporter was Ernest Lawrence. Oppenheimer's General Advisory Committee unanimously opposed the development of the H-bomb. Fermi and Rabi stated: "It is necessarily an evil thing considered in any light." President Truman was put under great pressure by the chairman of the Joint Congressional Committee on Atomic Energy, a member of the Atomic Energy Commission, and the Joint Chiefs of Staff to approve the H-bomb project, and in 1951 he directed the Los Alamos group to proceed. Teller returned to Los Alamos, but was unable to work effectively with his scientific colleagues. Thus, he and Ernest Lawrence campaigned successfully for the development of a second nuclear weapons laboratory, which eventually became the Lawrence Livermore Laboratory, in Livermore, California. In the climate of anti-Communist hysteria created by Senator Joseph McCarthy in the 1950s, Oppenheimer's patriotism was questioned, and he was deemed a security risk because of suspected Communist leanings.

Teller testified against Oppenheimer in government hearings

conducted in the 1950s to determine whether or not Oppenheimer should be given security clearance. He portrayed Oppenheimer and others who opposed the development of the H-bomb as unpatriotic and untrustworthy. Lord Zuckerman, strategic planning adviser to Air Marshal Tedder and General Eisenhower during World War II, wrote in 1988 that as a result of this testimony Teller was ostracized by the community of nuclear scientists. Rabi accused Teller of never "taking a position where there was the slightest chance in the interest of peace. I think he is an enemy of humanity."

During the 1950s the United States viewed the Soviet Union as the chief obstacle to international understanding. The policy of the U.S. government at that time with respect to collaborative efforts was to support freedom of access by the world's scientists to basic science laboratories involved in nuclear research. If the Soviet Union responded favorably to this first step, it might later be possible to move toward international control of nuclear energy. Narrow areas of agreement could be extended step by step as progress was attained. After an interchange of scientific knowledge, controls and safeguards could be developed without *prematurely* outlawing atomic weapons.

It was also U.S. government policy in the fifties to encourage the development of industrial uses of atomic energy, with mutual inspection of nuclear facilities, under the aegis of an international commission. All nations might be persuaded to agree to use nuclear fission exclusively for the production of electricity. No secret development of atomic weapons would be allowed. Existing bombs would be turned into fuel for power plants. The eventual control of nuclear weapons might even pave the way for eliminating conventional weapons and war itself.

Unfortunately, the worst fears of Leo Szilard, Admiral William Leahy, General George Marshall, and many others have come to pass: Whereas all the explosives detonated in World War II totaled two million tons of TNT, in 1988 the United States and the Soviet Union have nuclear weapons poised at each other that have the explosive power of 50 billion tons of TNT. Both nations are capable of launching an attack with atomic weapons that could kill hundreds of millions of people. As Jonathan Schell wrote in *The Fate of the Earth*, "What happened at Hiroshima was less than a millionth part of a holocaust at present levels of world nuclear armament. . . .

The totalities in question are now not single cities but nations, eco-systems, and the earth's ecosphere."

THE ATOMIC ENERGY ACT OF 1946

On August 12, 1946, the *General Account of the Development of Methods of Using Atomic Energy for Military Purposes*, the so-called Smyth report, was released to the American public. Its major recommendation was that the nation's atomic energy be transferred from military to civilian control. This proposal was the basis for one of the most significant pieces of legislation ever passed by the U.S. Congress: the Atomic Energy Act of 1946. By the time the act reached its final form and was passed, however, several critically important conclusions from the Smyth report had been dropped, namely: (1) it would be impossible to keep secret the methods of building nuclear weapons; (2) foreign nations would soon catch up with the United States in the development of nuclear weapons and the peaceful uses of atomic energy; (3) there was no effective defense against nuclear weapons; and (4) the destructive power of offensive weapons had far outstripped any nation's capacity to defend against them.

The authors of the Atomic Energy Act of 1946 accepted the fact that the misuse of atomic energy by design or through ignorance could "inflict incalculable disaster upon the nation, destroy the general welfare, imperil the national safety, and endanger world peace." They accepted the premise that government control and regulation of all aspects of atomic energy were imperative and that there should be full civilian, not military, control of nuclear weaponry.

The U.S. military did everything within its power to retain control of the development of nuclear weapons, but its efforts were thwarted. As is often the case in politics, chance events had enormous political consequences. On November 25, 1946, members of General Douglas MacArthur's occupation forces in Japan, acting on orders from Washington, dumped two Japanese cyclotrons into Tokyo Bay, despite the fact that these cyclotrons were of little military significance.

During the war, Yoshio Nishina, the foremost nuclear physicist in Japan, who had studied with Niels Bohr in Copenhagen before the war, had led a group of scientists in trying to determine whether it would be possible to build an atomic bomb for the Imperial Japanese Army. These scientists eventually gave up the effort and returned to other activities at Tokyo's Institute for Physical and Chemical Research, which was later severely damaged in April 1945 by an incendiary bomb. Nishina had directed the construction of two cyclotrons, one of them as large as one of Ernest Lawrence's in Berkeley, California. At the end of the war, for Nishina, the Japanese cyclotrons symbolized a postwar Japan that would reconstruct itself and fulfill its destiny despite great adversity. His goal was to help save the world by making Japan a mecca of international science and to prevent the destruction of the human species. After the U.S. Army's dumping of the Japanese cyclotrons into Tokyo Bay, Nishina's entire personality changed. He turned all his efforts toward the reindustrialization of Japanese science, and became vicechairman of the Japanese Science Council.

When news of the destruction of the Japanese cyclotrons was announced, many scientists in the United States strongly protested, citing this action as evidence that all aspects of nuclear energy should be under civilian control. In the process of transferring authority for developing and controlling nuclear weapons to civilian hands, the U.S. government directed the five-member U.S. Atomic Energy Commission (AEC) to develop and support a vigorous program of research that would disseminate the application of new discoveries about atomic energy to all interested persons. It also charged the commission with developing nonmilitary uses of nuclear energy and encouraging research by supplying fissionable material and radioactive isotopes free of charge to anyone who met the standards of personal safety and military security established by the AEC. In fact, the radioactive materials that were distributed according to the guidelines of the Atomic Energy Act of 1946 revolutionized biomedical research and medical practice by providing scientists all over the world with carbon-14, tritium (hydrogen-3), phosphorus-32, iodine-131, and, later, technetium-99m. These radioisotopes (usually referred to as "radionuclides") became major tools for biomedical research and health care, equaling in importance the invention of the microscope. They paved the way for the biomedical sciences to move from the cellular to the molecular level of organization.

3

NUCLEAR MEDICINE

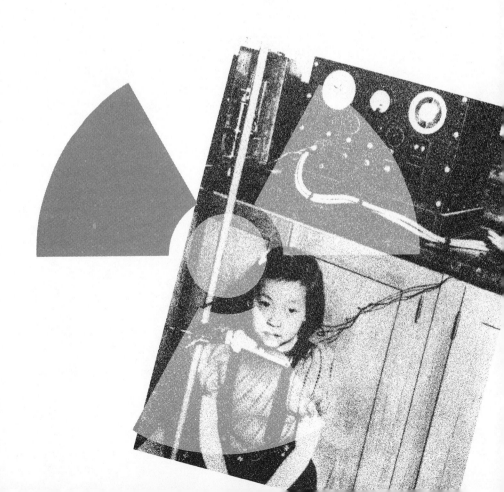

And then in a still more remote corner of this wing of the museum was revealed a collection of grapy, convoluted objects, stored in formalin to retard spoilage—shelf upon shelf of human brains. There must have been someone whose job it was to perform routine craniotomies on the cadavers of notables and extract their brains for the benefits of science.

Carl Sagan, Broca's Brain *(1979)*

Preceding page: Measurement of the accumulation of radioactive iodine by the thyroid gland with a Geiger-Müller detector, performed by Joseph Hamilton in Ernest Lawrence's laboratory in Berkeley, Calif., in 1941. Photograph from H. S. Taylor, E. O. Lawrence, and I. Langmuir, *Molecular Films: The Cyclotron and the New Biology* (New Brunswick, N.J.: Rutgers University Press, 1942). Reproduced by permission of the American Institute of Physics.

HOW IT BEGAN

The thermometer, chemical balance, and microscope served as the basis of scientific medicine for more than a century. With the introduction of the tracer principle by Hevesy, the discovery of artificial radioactivity by Joliot and Curie, and the invention of the cyclotron by Lawrence, it became possible to examine chemical reactions first in animals and then in human beings, and the field of biochemistry was born.

As set forth in the principle of the "dynamic state of body constituents," the entire body is a collection of many billions or trillions of dynamic chemical reactions. Even our bones, joints, and ligaments are continually being remolded to adjust to our bodily activities and weight. The cell was long considered the basic biological unit, but in studies using radioactive tracers, molecules have become a major focus as well, including their role in the communication that takes place among cells and organs. Hormones, enzymes, neurotransmitters, and receptors on cell surfaces control specific transport processes and are actively involved in transferring information from one cell to another.

In the late 1920s, Hermann Blumgart and Soma Weiss, two physicians at Massachusetts General Hospital, injected solutions of radium-C (bismuth-214, a naturally occurring radioactive material) into the veins of healthy persons and patients with heart disease to study the velocity of the circulating blood. These were the first applications of radioactive tracers in clinical research, and Blumgart eventually came to be known as the father of diagnostic nuclear medicine.

Today radioactive tracers play a major role not only in biomedical research but also in the care of millions of patients throughout the world. Three radionuclides—carbon-14, tritium (hydrogen-3), and phosphorus-32—remain the backbone of modern biomedical science, especially in the fields of biochemistry, molecular biology, and genetics. Biology, biochemistry, and medicine have made major advances as a result of the application of radioactive tracers.

The discovery of artificial radioactivity by Irène Curie and her husband, Frédéric Joliot, made it possible for Hevesy and other scientists to extend greatly the tracer principle. Joliot and Curie announced their scientific news in a short article in *Nature* on February 10, 1934: "Our latest experiments have shown a very striking fact: when an aluminum foil is irradiated by a polonium preparation, the emission of positrons does not cease immediately when the active preparation is removed. The foil remains radioactive and the emission of radiation decays exponentially as for an ordinary radioelement."

The discovery of artificial radioactivity opened the door for the production of radioactive tracers of practically every element, enabling investigators to tailor specific tracers for the study of specific biochemical processes. For example, by positioning a Geiger counter over a patient's neck, investigators discovered that the thyroid gland accumulates iodine-131 as iodide ions. Researchers also found that iodine metabolism is abnormal in patients with goiters. John Lawrence and Joseph Hamilton in Berkeley, and S. Hertz and A. Roberts in Boston, used radioiodine to diagnose patients whose thyroids were overactive (hyperthyroidism) or underactive (hypothyroidism). These findings paved the way for the administration of large doses of radioactive iodine to reduce the function of an overactive thyroid gland. Indeed, radioiodine therapy has become an alternative to surgery in the treatment of hyperthyroidism.

During the period 1943–1946, S. Seidlin, L. Marinelli, and E. Oshry began to use radioactive iodine-131 to treat patients with metastatic cancer of the thyroid. Metastases, even those located far from the thyroid, could be identified by searching the entire body with a Geiger counter shielded with lead in such a way as to give it directionality, a procedure called "radioisotope scanning." The news media in the late 1940s described dramatic cures of cancer of the thyroid following the administration of radioactive iodine-131, referring to the administered doses as "atomic cocktails." In those early days radioiodine was so expensive ($1,500 per dose) that after it was administered, it was recovered from a patient's urine for readministration to the patient. When reactor-produced radioiodine became available as a result of Enrico Fermi's invention of the nuclear reactor in 1941, the cost dropped to less than $100 per dose.

Radioactive phosphorus-32 selectively localizes in bone marrow, where its beta radiation can kill cancer cells. It was first used to treat a patient with chronic lymphatic leukemia on Christmas Eve, 1937, by John Lawrence, who had joined his brother Ernest Lawrence in founding the Donner Laboratory at the University of California in Berkeley. After Ernest invented the cyclotron, John decided to devote his professional life to the application of cyclotron-produced radioactive materials to medical diagnosis and treatment, and to the advancement of biomedical research. The Donner Laboratory was dedicated "to the application of physics, chemistry and the natural sciences to biology and medicine."

Phosphorus-32 soon gained wide acceptance in the treatment of blood diseases, a use that continues today for patients with polycythemia vera, a disease characterized by the overproduction of red blood cells. During and after World War II, phosphorus-32 was sent from Oak Ridge, Tennessee, to the University of California Medical School in Berkeley to treat patients with leukemia. The demand for radioactive materials, however, soon surpassed the limited supply provided by the nation's few extant cyclotrons.

The modern era of nuclear medicine began on June 14, 1946, when the prestigious journal *Science* announced that radioactive isotopes would be made available for public distribution from the Manhattan Project. The first shipment of a reactor-produced radioactive tracer to a civilian institution occurred on August 2, 1946, when carbon-14-labeled barium carbonate was sent to the Barnard Free Skin and Cancer Hospital in St. Louis, Missouri. It was a momentous event, and government officials and members of the press gathered in Oak Ridge to watch the shipment leave. Prior to its use in patients, carbon-14 carbonate was converted to carbon dioxide gas, and then into acetic acid, which was sent to Paul Rothenmund, of the Kettering Foundation, Antioch College, Ohio, for the production of the cancer-fighting drug carbon-14-methylcholanthrene.

These shipments were the first of a flood of radioisotopes sent all over the world from Oak Ridge, and later from Brookhaven National Laboratory, on Long Island, New York, another national laboratory established under the provisions of the Atomic Energy Act of 1946. Because of their access to the vast neutron-bombardment facilities that had been built during the war, these "national laboratories" (including Los Alamos National Laboratory and Argonne National Laboratory) began to issue "shopping lists" that grew in size every month, announcing new radionuclides available at cost for biomedical research and clinical applications. One item advertised on the cover of the 1960 Brookhaven catalog was technetium-99m, an isotope of an element that had not existed until Emilio Segrè and Glenn Seaborg produced it in 1938 using Ernest Lawrence's thirty-seven-inch cyclotron in Berkeley. This radionuclide languished on physicists' charts for more than two decades before it was recognized as having nearly ideal physical characteristics for studies of living human beings. Then it quickly became the most widely used radioactive tracer in *in vivo* nuclear medicine throughout the world as studies were undertaken in which radioactive substances called "radiopharmaceuticals" were administered to patients. Likewise, carbon-14 and tritium revolutionized *in vitro* biochemical research. Hardly a paper was published in biomedical science that did not report the use of one or the other of these radionuclides in the research.

On January 1, 1947, the responsibilities of the Manhattan District Project were transferred to the U.S. Atomic Energy Commission, in accordance with the Atomic Energy Act of 1946. Coming full circle, exactly ten years after the atomic bombing of Japan, the United States sent a traveling exhibition, the "Atoms for Peace Exhibition," to eight Japanese cities. The exhibit included displays of the various uses of atomic energy in medicine (cancer therapy, for instance), food preservation, the generation of electricity, and basic scientific research.

THE CHEMISTRY OF LIFE

Nuclear medicine is one of the most eclectic medical specialties because it incorporates the disciplines of nuclear physics, chemistry, electronics, engineering, physiology, and biochemistry into medicine. In the beginning, the field was called "atomic medicine." Essentially, it involves the measurement of radioactive tracers within the body using radiation detectors directed at the body from the outside (*in vivo* studies), and the measurement of radioactive tracers in body fluids such as blood and urine in the test tube (*in vitro* studies). The emission of gamma rays from radioactive tracers within the human body allows researchers to measure the regional function and biochemistry of practically every organ. Theoretically, whenever a physiological and biochemical process can be examined with radioactive tracers, at least two types of disease are possible: one in which the process takes place at an abnormally slow rate, and another in which the process is abnormally fast.

A nuclear medical procedure differs from an ordinary X-ray procedure in several ways. Most notably, in an X-ray procedure the radiation originates outside the body—from an X-ray machine—and is transmitted across the body to expose X-ray film. In a nuclear scanning procedure, small amounts of radioactive chemicals are injected into the patient's bloodstream, typically by way of an arm vein. Then the amount of radioactivity in different regions of the body or within an organ of interest is measured by means of externally placed radiation detectors, which count the number of photons coming from the patient. Selection of the specific radioactive tracer to be used depends on the particular bodily function or regional biochemical reaction that is to be studied.

In the early days of nuclear medicine, researchers prepared maps of regional function within organs such as the thyroid by laboriously counting point by point the radioactivity coming from the region of interest—the neck, for instance. By carefully charting activity levels, and joining points that had the same counts, investigators could draw "isocount" lines to form a picture of the distribution of the radioactive tracer within the region. Thus they were able to obtain crude pictures of organs which revealed anatomical detail and structural lesions such as tumors or abscesses. It then occurred to the American physicist Benedict Cassen that manual point-by-point counting could be eliminated by motorizing the radiation detector to move back and forth over the patients's body. The number of radioactivity "counts" measured by the detector could then be used to activate a moving pen, and the density of the ink dots subsequently recorded would be proportional to the amount of radioactivity measured from the different regions of the organ. Such dots provided an "image" of the relative number of radioactive disintegrations recorded from the area of the body being scanned.

In 1958, another American physicist, Hal Anger, invented a new method of imaging radioactivity distributed within the human body. He built the first scintillation camera, or "gamma camera," as it was later named. (The word *scintillation* refers to the flash of light that occurs in a crystal radiation detector when it is hit by a photon coming from the patient's body.) Using a pinhole to direct the gamma rays, Anger placed a bank of seven photomultiplier tubes against a large crystal radiation detector to amplify the weak signals coming from the light flashes in the crystal. The pattern of activation of the phototubes made it possible to locate where on the crystal the light flash had occurred when the gamma-ray photon hit the crystal. A computer then analyzed the pattern of recorded counts coming from the patient and converted them into an image of the distribution of the radioactive atoms within the patient's body. The "Anger camera" was made available commercially in 1964, and subsequently became the most commonly used instrument in nuclear medicine.

Today radioactivity can be measured with instruments sensitive enough to detect a single photon. This has made it possible to measure exceedingly low concentrations of chemical substances not only in body fluids such as blood but also within whole organs. In studies of various physiological processes, radioactive tracers that take part in specific chemical reactions in different organs of the body are administered to healthy persons and patients. The choice of the radioactive substance to be injected is determined by the chemical or physiological process to be examined. The movement of the tracer from one part of the body to another is measured, and the results are displayed as "scans" or "images" that reveal regional biochemistry.

Positron emission tomography (PET) uses radioactive atoms with a short half-life—that is, a rapid rate of radioactive decay, which keeps the radiation exposure of the patient within permissible limits and without side effects. The most common radionuclides used in PET scans are carbon-11 (half-life = 20 minutes), fluorine-18 (half-life = 110 minutes), and oxygen-15 (half-life = 2 minutes). These radionuclides, which emit positrons during the process of radioactive decay, are made in cyclotrons. The short half-life of carbon-11 makes it inconvenient to use in biochemistry; thus, the longer-lived radionuclide carbon-14, which can be produced in a nuclear reactor and at a lower cost, has rapidly replaced the short-lived carbon-11 for *in vitro* studies in laboratories throughout the world. Phosphorus-32 and tritium (hydrogen-3) also can be produced at a much lower cost in a reactor than in a cyclotron. The longer half-lives of carbon-14 and tritium make them ideal for *in vitro* biochemical studies, but they cannot be used to study regional chemistry in the living human body because they do not emit the types of penetrating radiation that can be picked up by radiation detectors outside the body. For that, one needs carbon-11.

The PET scanner consists of a ring of many small radiation detectors lining a large steel ring that surrounds the patient. It produces images of the distribution of the positron-emitting radiotracer at various times after the tracer's injection. When the scanner is used to measure glucose metabolism, the radionuclide fluorine-18 must be attached to deoxyglucose (an analog of glucose) molecules. After injection, the radioactively tagged (or labeled) deoxyglucose travels via the bloodstream throughout the body, including the brain, and behaves just like glucose, except that its metabolism stops at a certain point, almost like a freeze-frame photograph. Its distribution reveals the rate of glucose metabolism taking place within the region being examined.

The radioactivity from the fluorine-18-labeled deoxyglucose molecules can be measured because the fluorine-18 atoms emit positrons, which travel about one millimeter in all directions and then collide with electrons. Since the positron is antimatter and the electron is matter, this collision results in their mutual annihilation. The positron and electron disappear, and two gamma-ray photons are emitted in diametrically opposite directions from the body. The photons are of sufficiently high energy to travel from within the body to the outside, where they are measured by the ring of radiation detectors. PET "scans" or "images" are then constructed by a computer, which reveals the distribution of biochemical processes within the region of interest.

The PET scan, the CT (X-ray computed tomography) scan, the MRI (magnetic resonance imaging, previously called nuclear magnetic resonance, or NMR) scan, and the SPECT (single-photon emission computed tomography, another tool of nuclear medicine) scan all make use of the tomography principle—that is, they all obtain information from "slices" through the body—but where CT and MRI images reveal *structure,* PET and SPECT images reveal regional *chemistry.* The cross-sections, or "tomographic slices," of the distribution of radiotracers within the body that PET scans portray provide the same information that would be obtained if it were possible to remove slices from the patient's body and examine the chemical processes going on within the different regions.

The word *tomography* is derived from the Greek word *tomos,* meaning "a piece cut out, or a section." Each of the many tomographic slices corresponds to one section through the body. All the slices taken together provide a three-dimensional image of the body's chemistry. David Kuhl and his colleagues at the University of Pennsylvania were the first to develop tomographic images of radioactivity distributed within the brain, by means of a rotating array of radiation detectors. Nobel laureates G. Hounsfield and A. Cormack subsequently developed the CT scanner in the early 1970s, based on the use of computer science and the development of mathematical algorithms to reconstruct tomographic "slices" of the brain. In PET imaging, mathematical models are used to calculate regional concentrations of chemicals and reaction rates, which are then portrayed as images.

IMAGES OF BRAIN CHEMISTRY

As knowledge of neuroanatomy and neuropathology increased during the nineteenth century, physicians tried to relate mental symptoms to "organic" structural lesions. With the invention of the microscope, information about abnormal structure could be obtained at the cellular level. After World War II, radioactive tracers made it possible to examine the body at the molecular level, the domain of biochemistry.

In the 1950s the belief that mental diseases such as schizophrenia might be "organic" was strengthened by the finding that many of the symptoms of schizophrenia can be alleviated with drugs that have specific biochemical effects. Until that time, schizophrenia was thought to be caused by abnormal brain functioning resulting from stressful life experiences. The evidence that major mental diseases such as schizophrenia were associated with biochemical abnormalities of the brain, and that drugs could greatly relieve the symptoms of the disease, was supplemented by studies of body fluids and by the examination of patients' brains at autopsy. With the introduction of radioactive tracers it became possible to examine the chemistry of the living human brain, and to begin to relate the findings from these examinations to the mental aspects of thinking, feeling, and behavior.

Nuclear medicine brought about a whole new way of looking at disease by providing portraits of regional biochemical function within the organs of the living human being. Disturbed function within an organ such as the brain often results from structural abnormalities. Post-mortem examination at times reveals unmistakable anatomical abnormalities, and diseases, such as brain tumors, can produce almost every type of mental illness. In most cases of mental illness, however, anatomical changes cannot be detected even with the most advanced medical imaging systems, including X-ray computed tomography (CT) and magnetic resonance imaging (MRI), and we must turn to chemistry.

Radioactive tracers enable us to explore whether chemical abnormalities within the brain account for abnormal mental function and behavior, including delusions, hallucinations, thought disorder, and abnormal behavior. If reproducible abnormalities are found, diseases such as schizophrenia and manic-depressive illness may one day join pellagra, neurosyphilis, and other diseases manifesting biological correlates of mental dysfunction.

PET scans often reveal the presence of disease before anatomical changes show up on a CT scan. Since biochemical problems tend to occur before anatomical changes, PET scans can be used to diagnose disease at an earlier stage than was possible in the past.

With the PET scan, we can begin to decipher the "chemical language" of the brain—both in sickness and in health. We can measure the adequacy of the blood supply, the energy supply, and the chemical processes that transfer information among different regions of the brain. We have the tools to continue and expand the search for the biological bases of neurological and psychiatric disorders. Although most PET studies today are performed as part of research protocols, today's research is tomorrow's practice, just as today's practice was yesterday's research.

The PET scan also makes it possible for us to examine directly the effects of drugs on the chemistry of the brain, and is likely to improve the treatment of depression, epilepsy, Alzheimer's disease, drug and alcohol abuse, Parkinson's disease, and other disorders. For example, patients with Parkinson's disease have concentrations of the neurotransmitter dopamine that are 85 percent below normal in the parts of the brain involved with movement. Administering the amino acid L-dopa to these patients replenishes the supply of dopamine, and often greatly improves the patients' symptoms. By monitoring the responses of patients to specific types of drug treatment, researchers hope to increase the benefits of such treatment and to reduce the risk of untoward side effects from the drugs employed.

Nuclear medical techniques have already revealed characteristic patterns of regional blood flow and abnormal biochemical processes in the brains of patients with Alzheimer's disease, stroke, and the dementias associated with Parkinson's and Huntington's disease, as well as the location, severity, and extent of disease in patients with stroke, brain tumors, and epilepsy. One area in which PET imaging is moving into clinical practice is the treatment of epilepsy. Almost half of the approximately 800,000 Americans who have epilepsy do not respond adequately to drug treatment. Some of these patients would benefit from surgical therapy if the site in the brain from which the seizures originate, such as the temporal lobe, could be accurately identified. X-ray computed tomography and magnetic resonance imaging have the capacity to reveal structural abnormalities at this site in about 40 percent of epilepsy patients. Characteristic biochemical or blood-flow abnormalities detected by PET and SPECT are often found at the site from which the seizures originate.

Approximately 11,000–15,000 Americans develop primary brain tumors every year, with a resulting death rate of 4 per 100,000 persons. Modern nuclear medical techniques can be used to measure the metabolic activity of a tumor, which reflects its degree of malignancy; the more aggressive and dangerous a brain tumor is, the higher its metabolic rate. In addition, nuclear medical techniques can be used to delineate the extent of a brain tumor and to differentiate a tumor from the effects of radiation and other types of treatment, information that helps physicians plan and monitor treatment. Measurements of blood flow to a tumor, together with levels of glucose or oxygen consumption, are quantitative indicators of a patient's response to treatment.

In stroke patients, the abnormalities of regional glucose or oxygen metabolism detected by PET scans are often far more extensive than the corresponding anatomical changes detected by X-rays and CT scans. The patterns of these metabolic abnormalities correlate with the severity of the patients' symptoms, and help predict how much function they will eventually recover. Below a critical level, a reduction in blood flow to a given region of the brain results in a decrease in the supply of oxygen to that region, and can lead to irreversible brain damage. Regions in which oxygen metabolism has decreased but in which neurons are still alive can at times be helped by the administration of drugs or, in certain instances, by surgery to improve the blood flow to them. Nuclear medical techniques can distinguish the reversible from the irreversible effects of a stroke, which helps in planning treatment. PET scans have also been used to assess what types of treatment are helpful to stroke patients. Patients who have multiple small strokes sometimes develop dementia. The distribution of disease in these patients helps distinguish them from patients with another type of dementia—Alzheimer's disease.

Dementia patients fall into two broad categories: those who suffer from a disease process that can be halted or at times reversed, and those who can be treated only with supportive care. Thirty percent of demented elderly patients develop the condition as a result of impaired blood flow in the brain caused by blocked blood vessels. If such patients have high blood pressure, they can be treated. Another 20 percent of demented elderly patients can be treated by discontinuing medications that, singly or in combination, can cause dementia. Depression also is common in the elderly, and at times is accompanied by forgetfulness and confusion. If diagnosed correctly, depression can be treated successfully. Increased or decreased function of the thyroid gland and vitamin B12 deficiency are other causes of dementia that can be treated successfully if recognized. Blood clots involving the brain, resulting from unrecognized or minor trauma, can impair mental function. For all these reasons, diagnosis of the cause of dementia is important, but often may be difficult, especially in the early stages of the disease, when treatment can be most effective.

Half of all patients with dementia have Alzheimer's disease, which is usually diagnosed not directly but by excluding other possible causes of dementia. Because the disease is progressive, it is important for both the patient and the family that the diagnosis be made as early as possible. Clinical observations and psychological testing lead to a correct diagnosis of Alzheimer's disease in only half of all patients who first seek medical care because of memory loss. Often the diagnosis is made only after thousands of dollars have been spent on diagnostic tests in studies extending over many months. Brain scans involving radioactive tracers are beginning to provide information that facilitates the diagnosis of Alzheimer's disease well before it could be made with certainty on clinical grounds alone.

Alzheimer's disease is characterized by the abnormally accelerated death of nerve cells in certain regions of the brain. As a result of this neuronal degeneration, there is a secondary loss of blood flow and a decreased supply of oxygen and glucose to the involved regions of the brain. PET scans of patients with Alzheimer's disease show characteristically abnormal patterns of regional blood flow, glucose consumption, and oxygen metabolism, and these patterns make it possible to differentiate this disease from other forms of dementia, such as those associated with hydrocephalus or stroke.

Because of its ability to measure chemical reactions in the brain, the PET scan also allows researchers to study schizophrenia. Both electrical and chemical changes transmit information throughout the brain and the rest of the nervous system. How each of us perceives the outside world is reflected in the electrochemistry of our brain. Chemicals secreted into different regions of the brain affect our emotions, our thinking, and our behavior, and probably help encode our memories.

Before the introduction of the PET scan, studies of brain chemistry were limited to experimental animals or examination of the human brain at autopsy. Such studies revealed the existence of neuroreceptors, chemical "recognition sites" within the brain that direct the transmission of signals from one neuron to another or from a neuron to a muscle or a gland. Put more simply, these neuroreceptors guide the brain in responding to the wealth of sensory inputs it receives from the outside world. With the PET scan, it is now possible for researchers to study neuroreceptors in living human beings and to relate their findings to patterns of human behavior.

The first successful PET imaging of a neuroreceptor in the brain of a living human being was achieved on May 25, 1983, following the injection of a carbon-11-labeled drug, N-methylspiperone, which binds to dopamine receptors. Most dopamine receptors are located in the groups of nerve cells (or neurons) found at the base of the brain, the caudate nucleus and the putamen, the regions involved with movement and emotion. PET scans have since revealed that dopamine receptors in normal human beings decrease by almost 50 percent between the ages of nineteen and seventy-three years, with most of the decrease occurring before the age of forty.

More than twenty years ago, A. Carlsson, of the University of Göteborg, Sweden, first proposed that dopamine metabolism of the brain might be abnormal in patients with schizophrenia, a disease characterized by delusions, hallucinations, disordered thinking, withdrawal from society, and a lack of emotional responsiveness, motivation, and identity. Carlsson based his idea on the finding that dopamine receptors are blocked by drugs that help schizophrenic patients. Amphetamines, which elevate dopamine concentrations within neurons, exacerbate the symptoms in schizophrenic patients and produce psychotic states resembling schizophrenia in normal persons. Postmortem studies of the brains of some schizophrenic patients revealed increased numbers of dopamine receptors in the caudate nucleus and putamen. In many cases researchers could not determine whether the increase in the number of receptors was a compensatory response to the patients' having been treated in the past with drugs that block dopamine receptors or whether the increase was an intrinsic part of the disease.

Recent PET studies by Dean Wong and a team of researchers at the Johns Hopkins University revealed that there are nearly twice as many dopamine receptors in the caudate nucleus and putamen of some patients with schizophrenia—even in patients who have never received receptor-blocking drugs—than in normal persons. It is not known whether the increase in the number of dopamine receptors precedes or follows the onset of symptoms of schizophrenia. Elevated receptor concentrations could result from a decrease in the quantity of dopamine in the involved neurons. Dopamine levels may be high early in the disease but subsequently decrease, with a resultant increase in receptors. Wong and his associates also found an elevated number of dopamine receptors in some depressed patients with psychotic symptoms.

In addition to helping explore the mechanisms of mental disorders, PET imaging and other techniques involving positron-emitting tracers can be used to examine the effects of drugs on the brain. German bacteriologist Paul Ehrlich postulated at the turn of this century that the effects of drugs on the body might be explained by a chemical binding that occurs between drugs and specific chemical groups on cell surfaces called "receptors." Three decades ago an extract of an Indian herb, *Rauwolfia serpentina*, proved helpful in the treatment of high blood pressure. What was remarkable was that the drug had a calming effect without sedation in hypertensive patients who also suffered from schizophrenia. This unexpected discovery was the forerunner of the modern drug treatment of mental disorders. Researchers later found that reserpine was the component of the herb that was affecting the process of chemical neurotransmission.

The discovery of other drugs with similar effects soon followed, and some of these drugs reduced the concentration of chemical neurotransmitters within the brain—dopamine and norepinephrine, for instance. The drugs that were effective in treating patients with schizophrenia blocked the binding of dopamine to the brain's dopamine receptors, thereby inhibiting their neuronal activity. Another milestone was the discovery in 1965 that patients with Parkinson's disease had low dopamine concentrations in areas of the brain that control movement and emotion. This finding eventually led to the discovery that oral administration of the amino acid L-dopa to patients with Parkinson's disease relieved many of their symptoms, and thus further evidence was gained of the link between brain chemistry and behavior.

Measuring brain chemistry with positron-emitting radiotracers makes it possible for researchers to monitor the effects of drugs— both legal and illicit—on the human brain and to relate the chemical effects of drugs to their subjective effects. Planning and monitoring the drug treatment prescribed for psychiatric disorders may soon routinely involve monitoring the effects of drugs on brain chemistry as well as clinically assessing the effects of drugs on the patient's symptoms. Both PET scanning and a newly developed, simpler, much less expensive radiation-detection system have been used for this purpose.

It is hard to imagine physicians treating patients for hypertension without measuring their blood pressure—that is, relying only on the patients' symptoms as a guide to treatment. Yet that is how psychiatrists and other physicians have prescribed psychoactive drugs for the treatment of mental disorders. In the future, clinicians may be able to use PET or simpler radiation-detection devices to select appropriate drugs and to assess their patients' biochemical as well as behavioral responses to treatment.

One of the greatest benefits of PET imaging lies in its potential for testing directly the hypothesis that mental illnesses such as schizophrenia and depression are related to measurable abnormalities in brain chemistry. Of equal importance is the new technology's potential for advancing the science of "normal" human behavior as well as our understanding of why people act in undesirable ways under certain circumstances. It may well be that violence and destructive behavior are related to chemical changes in the brain, and, if so, they may someday come to be considered the manifestations of disease rather than willful misconduct.

THE CHEMISTRY OF HUMAN DESTRUCTIVENESS

Stellar dust and gas—from which all life on earth developed—eventually evolved into creatures who were able to think, feel, and act—that is, exercise the functions of the mind. For centuries, philosophers and scientists have tried to connect the workings of the mind to the brain—the most complex concentration of matter and energy on earth. Perhaps the greatest frontier of modern times is the search for the physicochemical correlates of consciousness, memory, reason, instincts, passions, and appetites—in short, an understanding of how chemical and electrical energy is transformed into human thoughts and emotions. The most fundamental question of mind/brain science is the nature of consciousness. An important practical question is why human behavior is so often violent and destructive.

According to the French philosopher Henri Bergson, "We *think* with only a small part of our past, but it is with our entire past that we desire, will, and act." Conscious thought is only the tip of the iceberg; our experiences and memories have an even greater influence on our behavioral responses to the external environment. The richer the experiences and memories, the greater the variety of possible responses. Bergson defined *consciousness* as the process of thinking about alternative behaviors when faced with external stimuli: "Consciousness seems proportionate to the living being's power of choice. Consciousness lights up the potentialities that surround an act. It fills the interval between what is done and what might be done."

Ionian philosophers in prehistoric Greece thought that water, earth, air, and fire—having the physical qualities of wet, dry, cold, and warm—were the primordial elements of being. From cold, dry earth, cold, wet water, hot, dry fire, and warm, moist air came the permutations and combinations of the humors: hot, moist blood; cold, moist phlegm; hot, dry (yellow) bile; and cold, dry (black) bile. Millennia later, in the eighteenth century, the concept of "internal secretions" of humors was revived by Theophile de Bordeu, a Parisian physician who maintained that each organ elaborated a specific product that passed into the blood. A century later, the great chemist Emil Fischer, working in Berlin, founded the science of biochemistry when he discovered the structure of carbohydrates and proteins, the chemical compounds that are peculiarly characteristic of all living processes. Today it is well known that the thyroids, parathyroids, hypophysis, pancreas, adrenals, and gonads produce chemical substances called "hormones," and that when secreted into the bloodstream, these hormones play a major role in regulating body chemistry and affecting behavior. In the last two decades, it has become increasingly clear that chemicals also play a major role in the functions of the nervous system.

Today it is possible to examine these chemicals within the living human brain and to begin to relate chemical events to human behavior. One view of the brain is that of psychiatrists, psychologists, sociologists, and others, who view the brain "from above," from the study of human behavior. Until now, the study of the brain "from below" has been the domain of more basic neuroscientists, who have examined the electrical and molecular changes occurring in isolated neurons of experimental animals. New medical imaging techniques, especially the PET scan, now make it possible for researchers to connect these two approaches. The human passions of threatening and aggressive behavior, as well as loving behavior, may one day be found to be reflected in the chemistry of the brain, in the patterns and amounts of hormones, neurotransmitters, and neuroreceptors found within different regions of the brain.

It may be that while our thoughts originate in our perception of the rapidly changing events in our external environment, our reactions to these events are determined in part by the combination of the incoming data with "recognition sites"—that is, enzymes and neuroreceptors within the brain. A reasonable hypothesis is that we are born with a set of recognition sites that we inherit from our parents and from generations of ancestors, and that our life experiences then continuously modify these sites. It is now possible to test this hypothesis by examining directly in the living human brain the types, numbers, and states of the neuroreceptors found there.

Consider for a moment the effects of drugs on brain chemistry. For better or worse, there is no question that our thoughts, feelings, and behavior are affected by drugs. Drugs have been used for millennia to relieve pain and misery, or, when abused, to increase human misery and destructiveness. Today, practically everyone takes psychoactive drugs in one form or another—for example, nicotine, alcohol, and caffeine. As people have become more anxious or lonely and psychoactive drugs have become more readily available, the use of such drugs has increased. The statistics on the abuse and devastating effects of licit and illicit psychoactive drugs document the increasing incidence of psychological and physical dependence, addiction, and violent or criminal activities. Every day in the United States, out of a population of 244 million, 1,000 people die as a result of smoking, 350 die from the effects of alcohol, 10 die after taking stimulant drugs (such as cocaine and codeine), 4–18 die from overdoses of sedatives and antidepressants, 4–12 die from the effects of narcotics, and a few die as a result of ingesting hallucinogens and tranquilizers. Smoking marijuana contributes to impaired performance. Take, for example, the fatal accident near Baltimore, Maryland, in which a freight train failed to stop at signals and moved into the path of a passenger train, thereby killing 16 people. The engineer of the freight train was later found to be a marijuana user.

In the United States today, 5 percent of senior high school students drink alcoholic beverages daily (down from 7 percent in the 1970s). Four percent smoke marijuana at least twenty times per month (down from 10 percent in the 1970s). Eight percent of young adults take cocaine. In a nationwide survey, 23 million people admitted that they had taken illegal drugs within the preceding thirty days.

Each year, more than 7 million adults abuse alcohol to the point of severe consequences, including loss of jobs, arrest, or illness. In 1980, alcohol abuse was often the cause of death: 9,200 deaths due to alcoholic liver disease (cirrhosis); 7,300 deaths from cancer; 50 percent of the deaths in 52,000 motor vehicle accidents; 30 percent of the suicides and 50 percent of the homicides, which accounted for 20,000 deaths. The total economic cost of alcohol abuse in the United States was estimated to be $89 billion in 1980 and $117 billion in 1983.

Today alcoholism is classified as a disease rather than as willful misconduct. Biological factors are now believed to play an important role. A genetic factor is suggested by the fact that the risk of becoming an alcoholic is three to five times greater for a person who has an alcoholic parent. Alcoholism also seems to be related to aggressive behavior. Data on boys studied from the first grade through later life indicate that aggressive behavior, especially when accompanied by shyness, increases by a factor of two or three the risk that problems with alcohol will develop later in life.

Alcohol and other drugs, both licit and illicit, affect the chemical reactions that take place at neuronal synapses, the contact points or "bridges" at which information is transmitted from one neuron to another. Each of the 30 billion neurons within the human brain has synaptic connections with about 10,000 other neurons. Drugs and the body's own chemical messengers, called "neurotransmitters," act at these synapses. Hundreds of different neurotransmitters, including more than fifty small molecules, such as norepinephrine and dopamine, and more than seventy larger molecules, called "neuropeptides," such as the naturally occurring opiates, carry information and affect behavior. Some drugs act by stimulating the release of neurotransmitters into the synapses; others, by blocking the interaction of the body's neurotransmitters with neuroreceptors; others, by interfering with the enzymes that break down the neurotransmitters after they have carried out their function of binding to postsynaptic receptors. Still others block the recycling of the neurotransmitters back into the presynaptic neurons from which they were originally secreted, only to be released again as a result of new electrical nerve impulses coming down the presynaptic axons.

Currently, radioactive tracer molecules are being used in experiments designed to find out what stimulates or inhibits the secretion of different neurotransmitters into different regions of the brain. A major effort is also being made to find out how sensory stimulation and behavior affect the types and numbers of neuroreceptors found in those regions. The chemicals released in the brain of a man while he is taking a romantic stroll down a country lane may be quite different from those secreted by a man who is searching for a victim to mug in an urban slum. It may someday be possible to relate certain types of behavior to chemical changes in the brain. Characteristic changes in brain chemistry may be associated with aggressive or violent behavior. Perhaps even viewing violence on television or in "splatter and slasher" movies may bring about measurable changes in brain chemistry.

PET imaging makes it possible to explore the unconscious as well as the conscious mind. The chemistry of aggression may be manifest at conscious, partially conscious, or even unconscious levels. In any case, aggression is well established in the human psyche. We cannot look at medieval torture devices in museums and reassure ourselves that we are less cruel today than people were hundreds of years ago. Survivors of Hitler's concentration camps and the Khmer Rouge's genocide in Cambodia walk among us. Amnesty International documents daily instances of unspeakable torture in countries on every continent and in every political system. Many sporting events are remnants of barbaric fighting rituals. The difference between Roman gladiators and modern professional football players in the United States is one of degree.

Ethologists K. Lorenz, R. Audry, and others conceived of aggression as innate, biologically adaptive impulses that serve to increase the chances of survival of the individual and the species. According to this view, wars are caused by an inherent destructive trend in human nature. Freud proposed that the innate passion to destroy, the death instinct, is equal in strength to the passion to love, the love instinct. His thesis was that the human race's aggressive behavior is the basic cause of war, crime, and personal quarrels, and that all kinds of destructive and sadistic behavior result from genetically programmed instincts. Among the important questions to be addressed by PET imaging is whether brain chemistry can be modified by environmental factors or is set in characteristic patterns at, or soon after, birth.

During the 1960s and 1970s, attention shifted toward socioeconomic factors, such as poverty and lack of education, as important contributors to aggressiveness or criminal behavior. Today the pendulum swings back and forth in the "nurture versus nature" debate as more new information is brought to light. The question remains whether environment or heredity is the main cause of aggressive human behavior. With PET imaging, we can begin to explore the degree to which biological and social factors affect brain chemistry. Perhaps one day we will speak of an individual's brain *chemotype* as well as his or her genotype and phenotype.

BENEFITS VERSUS RISKS

Since the late 1940s and early 1950s, physicians and scientists have been trained to understand and to handle and administer radioactive tracers safely. A basic course was established in 1947 that is still taught today at the Oak Ridge Institute of Nuclear Studies (now called the Oak Ridge Associated Universities). Consideration of the health hazards associated with ionizing radiation led to the development of a new scientific discipline called "health physics," which addresses the problems of protecting nuclear workers, patients, and the general public. The radiation safety officer in a hospital, laboratory, or company that handles radioactive materials is often a health physicist.

Throughout history, military-oriented research has made major contributions to human well-being, the development of penicillin being one example and nuclear medicine another. The development of the atomic bomb helped pave the way for nuclear medicine. Without a doubt, if the United States had not needed uranium, the nuclear reactor at Oak Ridge—which eventually supplied a plethora of radioactive isotopes for use in biochemical experiments and nuclear medicine—would never have been built.

Some would argue that counting the number of people who

have been helped by nuclear medicine should help reduce feelings of guilt and sorrow over the development of nuclear weapons. Others would say that the subsequent application of atomic energy to medicine in no way justified the creation of atomic weapons at the end of World War II. Regardless of one's viewpoint, the truth is that the human effort and resources devoted to the Manhattan Project and the subsequent transfer of that technology to peaceful uses of the atom have contributed greatly to human welfare. It makes one wonder how much more might be accomplished if the funds now used worldwide to produce and maintain nuclear weapons were used instead in the fields of biomedical research, health care, and other peaceful applications of atomic energy.

We are so awed and horrified by the destructive power of nuclear weapons that we forget that war itself—all kinds—is what we should abhor and prevent, not just nuclear war. We need to realize that the roots of war lie not only in politics, economics, and diplomacy but also, and perhaps even more importantly, in fear, aggression, and violent behavior. During Lyndon B. Johnson's presidential election campaign of 1964, a controversial television advertisement showed a little girl plucking daisy petals as she recited, "He loves me. He loves me not." She stared straight ahead as the camera zoomed in on her eyes, and the eerie whistling of a falling bomb was heard in the background. The viewer seemed to be staring into her mind as the pupil of her eye exploded into a mushroom cloud. When the noise died down, a calm man's voice stated, "We must learn to love one another if we are to live together." The message is still timely. Today, new medical technologies, particularly PET imaging, can help us learn more about the fear, aggression, and violence that are so deeply ingrained in the human psyche. If we succeed in relating the chemistry of the brain to certain aspects of normal and abnormal behavior, we may be able to reduce the threat to all mankind not only from nuclear warheads but also from conventional weapons.

4

LIVING WITH
UNCERTAINTY

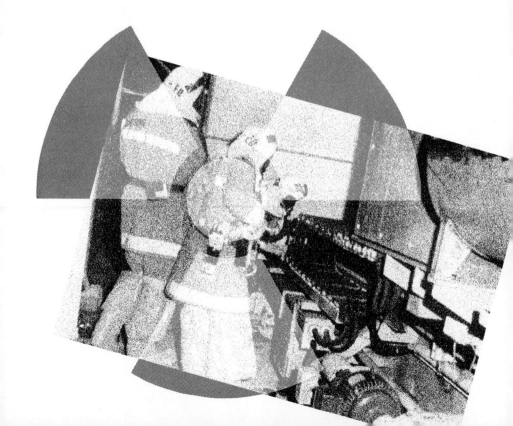

What do I fear? Myself? There's none else by.

Shakespeare, Richard III

RADIATION AND WOMEN

Was it fear or aggression that led Admiral Hyman Rickover to prohibit women from entering nuclear submarines or any other radiation area? Was Rickover right to believe that women are more likely than men to be damaged by ionizing radiation? During the 1920s, young women in New Jersey and Illinois were hired to paint a radium-laced substance on the dials of luminous clocks and watches. These women were paid according to the number of pieces they painted, and to increase their output, they sharpened the tips of their brushes by twirling them between their lips. In doing so, they inadvertently ingested large amounts of radium-226 and radium-228, which accumulated in their bones and resulted in cancer years later.

Today, there are no occupations from which women may be excluded because of radiation hazards. Women work in many occupations involving radiation, including naval and civilian nuclear reactor engineering, health physics, radiochemistry, radiology, nuclear medicine, nuclear medical technology, and X-ray technology. Women make up more than half of the 1 million people in the United States who in their workplaces are exposed to levels of ionizing radiation that are higher than background. Of these, 75 percent are involved in health care; the remainder are employed in industry or government. Of every 100,000 women of childbearing age in the United States, about 7,000 are pregnant at any one time; among radiation workers, the number is close to 42,000. Has the increase in the number of women in workplaces involving radiation been a step in the direction of greater economic freedom for women or a failure to recognize special risks? Should pregnant women be prevented from working with ionizing radiation?

Should a woman have a mammogram as a diagnostic test for breast cancer every year, or does the risk of radiation outweigh the benefits? Is a woman exposed to a radiation hazard every time she uses a video display terminal or a microwave oven, or when her baggage goes through an X-ray fluoroscopic machine at an airport? How is a woman to decide whether or not she is being exposed to unacceptable amounts of ionizing radiation?

The first step in answering these questions is to distinguish between *perceived* risk and *actual* risk. In issues involving radiation, the perception of risk is often much greater than the real risk, for many reasons:

1. People feel uncomfortable, insecure, and anxious when faced with complex subjects, and tend to oversimplify issues or jump to conclusions. They focus on one factor to the exclusion of other, equally important factors.
2. People are not yet used to dealing with uncertainty and risk, especially in quantitative terms. They go about their daily activities, not dwelling on the fact that many entail significant risk. When they are conscious of risk, they often insist that the risk be zero; that way, they redefine the activity as safe.
3. People are confused by conflicting reports by experts. They can't judge correctly the qualifications of experts, or detect fallacies in scientific arguments or omissions in scientific evidence. They may fail to recognize conflicts of interest on the part of experts. They may place unwarranted trust in scientists who have become media experts as a result of frequent appearances.

For example, in November 1981, television personality Phil Donahue interviewed John W. Gofman, a nuclear scientist and the author of the widely read book *Radiation and Human Health*. Between 1947 and 1963, Gofman led a team of scientists at the Lawrence Radiation Laboratory in California in the discovery of fat-carrying proteins (lipoproteins) in blood, using the newly invented ultracentrifuge. Their results were of great importance in revealing the relationship between dietary fats and coronary heart disease. Gofman's work eventually led to a decrease in fat consumption in the United States, which has played a role in the decline in coronary heart disease. Unfortunately, at the time of Gofman's original report of his results, his work was not accepted by his scientific peers. This so distressed him that in 1963 he left the laboratory and became a commercial fisherman for three years. When he returned to work as a scientist, he began to study the biological effects of low-level radiation. Again, however, his results were not well received by the scientific community, and again he left the laboratory. Since that time, he has often taken public positions opposing the use of radiation in medicine and industry. For example, he has claimed that every year in the United States more than 1.5 million people die as a result of unnecessary medical radiation. On the Donahue Show, Gofman stated that medical radiation poses a "major health hazard and causes cancer." Physicians reported that many of their female patients refused to have mammograms after seeing the show. This example illustrates how perceived risk can differ from real risk.

Breast cancer is the most common form of cancer in women and is second only to lung cancer as the cause of death from cancer in women. In 1987, approximately 130,000 new cases of invasive, and 5,000 cases of highly localized, breast cancer were diagnosed in the United States. Approximately 35 percent, or 45,000, of the women with invasive breast cancer are expected to die of the disease. Mammography is currently the most effective method of detecting breast cancer; it extends, but does not replace, periodic self-examination and examination by a physician. Much harm can result from an exaggerated perception of the risk of mammography. There is strong evidence that deaths from breast cancer in women can be reduced significantly if mammographic screening is carried out on a regular basis in women after the age of fifty. The evidence for reduction in mortality is not as clear-cut for women between the ages of forty and forty-nine.

In 1982, Lauriston Taylor, an expert in radiation measurements and protection for more than sixty years, published an article in the August issue of the *Health Physics Society Newsletter*, pointing out major inaccuracies of John Gofman's claims. For example, the Donahue Show had displayed an excerpt from Gofman's book stating that official estimates of the hazards to the public from radiation are too low by a factor of fifty. According to Taylor, the radiation protection standards that have been in use throughout the world for the past forty years have overestimated, not underestimated, the risks of radiation.

Mammography is the best example of the effective use of ionizing radiation for the detection of cancer early, for it does so at a stage when cure rates of 90 percent are possible. The procedure detects tumors that are too small to be felt by the patient or the physician. About 1 million women who have had breast cancer are still alive, and there is reason for optimism. Today 90 percent of women with breast cancer survive for at least five years after the initial diagnosis. A survey by the American Cancer Society and the National Cancer Institute involving 280,000 women showed that mammography on a regular basis resulted in 81 percent of the patients' being alive eight years after diagnosis. It is true that a decade ago mammography delivered a dose of radiation that may have increased the risk of cancer, but this problem has been solved by the introduction of equipment that provides a much lower dose of radiation. The American Cancer Society recommends that all women between the ages of thirty-five and thirty-nine have a "baseline" mammogram, and then have one every other year until the age of fifty, after which the procedure should be repeated every year. Women with a family history of breast cancer should have a mammogram every year, beginning at the age of thirty-five. Because women frequently have their mammograms taken at different facilities, they are advised to obtain their own copies of the studies to facilitate comparisons at later dates.

What about pregnant radiation workers? Exposure of the fetus to radiation is particularly harmful between the second and seventh weeks of pregnancy, when the organs are rapidly developing. A pregnant woman should limit her exposure to ionizing radiation to one-tenth the whole-body exposure level that is acceptable for nonpregnant radiation workers. A pregnant woman should undergo diagnostic X-rays or nuclear medical tests only if such studies are likely to influence decisions about the care of medical conditions complicating the pregnancy or unrelated to the pregnancy, but the procedures should be deferred until after the pregnancy if at all possible. Congenital abnormalities (teratogenesis) result from doses of radiation that are far higher than one would receive in diagnostic X-rays or nuclear medical procedures. In every case, proper technique in the performance of such procedures is mandatory to ensure that all exposure to radiation, including medical radiation, during pregnancy is kept as low as possible.

The Food and Drug Administration's standards for X-ray machines, in effect since 1974, cover technical requirements, such as automatically keeping the size of the X-ray beam the same as the size of the X-ray film being used. Nevertheless, instrument design can go only so far in minimizing the radiation dose received from X-ray examinations. The X-ray technician who performs the examination must be certain that the film size is appropriate for the region being examined. For example, when examining an infant's kidneys, the X-ray technician should manually override the machine's automatic system so that the size of the beam is smaller than the size of the film.

Shielding is another method used to reduce unnecessary radiation exposure during X-ray procedures. The reproductive organs in both women and men should be shielded with lead in examinations of the pelvis and lower back, as long as this can be accomplished without obscuring the region under diagnostic study. Developing the X-ray films properly is another way to decrease the patient's exposure to radiation. An overexposed X-ray film means an overexposed patient.

Motivation, education of health professionals and the public, and better communication are important in eliminating unnecessary exposure to radiation. Education of the patient (or parent) is the key. A sprained ankle, especially in a child, usually results in a trip to the physician or hospital to "get an X-ray to make sure that nothing is broken." People like the reassurance that a normal X-ray provides. After a bad fall, they don't say "I'm going to have a doctor check my ankle." They say, "I'm going to get my ankle X-rayed." Fortunately, X-ray procedures that were routine in the past, including the chest X-ray on admission to a hospital for whatever cause, are being eliminated. Unfortunately, the threat of malpractice may influence these decisions.

The best way to reduce exposure is not to have any examinations involving ionizing radiation, either X-rays or nuclear medical procedures, unless they are needed for diagnosis or treatment. Patients should not hesitate to ask their doctors why a particular X-ray procedure is needed. Such a dialogue lets the doctor know that his or her patient, or the patient's parent, is aware of the potentially harmful effects of X-rays. The doctor will then know that the patient does not need the reassurance associated with having "had an X-ray."

The following guidelines can help keep an individual's exposure to radiation to a minimum:

1. Ask the doctor why the X-ray is needed. Will it influence future treatment or the medical outcome?
2. Don't insist on an X-ray procedure, either directly or subtly.
3. Don't refuse an X-ray procedure because of fear of harmful effects of ionizing radiation. Often, not having an X-ray is much more harmful than the risk of the radiation.
4. Tell the physician and technician if you are or might be pregnant. They will usually ask. If they don't, tell them. This is especially important in the first trimester of pregnancy.
5. Ask for lead shielding of the reproductive organs if they are to be in the direct X-ray beam, but be aware that in some cases such shielding can't be used.
6. Keep a record of your X-ray examinations, including when and what kind of X-rays were taken. Retrieving previous X-rays can sometimes eliminate the need to repeat them, or can provide the doctor with important information about the progress of a disease.

What about the health effects of video display terminals (VDTs)? Increasingly, the public has expressed concern over possible adverse health effects, ranging from muscle strain to eye damage, birth defects, emotional stress, and angina. Various organized groups and individuals, including Dr. Rosalie Bertell, referred to previously, have advocated legislation affecting the use of VDTs in the workplace, including mandatory job rotation, avoidance of such work during pregnancy, and routine medical examinations. Possible radiation effects from VDTs came to the attention of the public in 1977, when cataracts were found in several employees of the *New York Times*. In 1979, malformed infants were born to four women who had been VDT operators during their pregnancies; the reports of these birth defects generated considerable anxiety. The concern resulted from the fact that certain brands of color television sets manufactured before 1970 emitted X-rays. That is no longer the case, and extensive studies have determined that radiation levels associated with VDTs are in the very low range of 0.2 mrems per year. No association has been found between prolonged use of VDTs and the incidence of abortions, birth defects, or cataracts. In the United States, legislation dealing with these issues is pending in at least eighteen states, despite the large body of scientific data which indicates that no radiation hazard is associated with even prolonged use of VDTs on a regular basis.

RESURGENT FEAR

In the spring of 1986, just as the Three Mile Island nuclear accident of 1979 was becoming a distant memory, disaster struck in the Soviet Union, evoking the frightening, almost apocalyptic image of technology gone berserk. To opponents of nuclear energy, the events at Three Mile Island and Chernobyl proved conclusively that nuclear power poses a far greater threat to public health than does a shortage of energy. They believe that all nuclear reactors are too dangerous and should be shut down as quickly as possible. In New England, the Clamshell Alliance has as its goal "to oppose nuclear power in all its forms." The position of Massachusetts governor Michael Dukakis on September 9, 1987, was that "since there is no known way to safely dispose of nuclear waste, the Governor opposes licensing of any new nuclear power plant."

Proponents of nuclear power believe that the Three Mile Island accident proved how well containment buildings and other safety features at well-designed nuclear facilities work, even in the face of serious human errors that are capable of causing injurious radiation exposure to both power plant employees and the general public. They view the Chernobyl disaster in 1986, which produced the first casualties from nonmilitary-oriented nuclear power, as a careless accident that occurred within an obsolete type of nuclear reactor that is not used to generate electricity in the Western world. They believe that a Chernobyl-type accident could never happen at a commercial nuclear power plant in the United States or in any other Western country.

The Chernobyl accident was a major industrial disaster that caused 31 deaths and forced the evacuation of 135,000 people within a 30-kilometer radius of the nuclear reactor. Review of the events leading up to the accidents at Three Mile Island and Chernobyl can tell us how accidents happen, and what we should do to prevent them or respond to them when they occur (which, given enough time, is inevitable).

Three Mile Island

In the early morning of March 28, 1979, Unit 2, a brand-new second-generation pressurized-water nuclear reactor located on Three Mile Island, in the middle of the Susquehanna River, in rural Pennsylvania, was humming along, generating nearly 1,000 megawatts of electricity for customers in southeastern Pennsylvania and New Jersey. Ordered in 1968, the reactor was a $750 million showpiece built by the Babcock and Wilcox Company, and had been in operation at full power for only three months.

During the previous year, only two new nuclear power plants had been ordered in the United States, down from a high of forty-one orders in 1973. The reasons for the declining interest were the escalation of the costs of building the plants, high interest rates, procedural and regulatory delays related to licensing, a fall in the demand for electricity, financial problems exacerbated by the economic recession from 1975 onward, and increasing opposition from antinuclear movements and environmental groups, including Friends of the Earth, the Sierra Club, and the Green Party (in Germany). (All orders for nuclear power plants placed between 1974 and 1978 have since been canceled, and none have been placed since 1978.)

In a reactor of the Three Mile Island type, the water system surrounding the core of the reactor is kept at high pressure to prevent the formation of steam even at the high temperatures produced by the reactor. Heat is transferred from the primary water system surrounding the core to the steam generator, which drives the turbines to generate electricity.

A few minutes before 4:00 A.M. on March 28, 1979, workers in the basement of the turbine building were replenishing resin columns used to purify the water inside the steam generator that drove the turbines that produced electricity. In the process, a backflow of water from the resin beds accidentally switched off a pump used to return the condensed steam after it had passed through the turbine. This immediately led to an automatic shutdown of the reactor, and activated auxiliary feedwater pumps to keep the steam generator from overheating.

These types of problems were routine, and were well taken care of by automatic control mechanisms. In nuclear power plants, multiple pumps are used to ensure a continuous flow of water throughout the system to prevent overheating. In an emergency, the reactor can be shut down by insertion of control rods to stop the nuclear reactions, but even after this has been done, the water flow must be maintained because heat continues to be generated, heat that is equal to about 6 percent of the full power of the reactor.

As is usually the case in a serious accident, several errors occurred at the Three Mile Island plant. Taken individually, each could easily have been taken care of, but occurring together, these errors led to disaster. Problems had begun several days earlier, when a valve connecting one of the auxiliary pumps that had been manually closed during a test of the pumps was not reopened. Because this valve was shut, the automatically activated auxiliary pumps were unable to supply enough cooling water. Excessive heat developed in the primary cooling water, which increased the volume of that water. This caused a rise in the water level in a water-filled pressurizer that automatically adjusts the pressure in the primary cooling system. All of the above-mentioned events, plus the automatic insertion of control rods to stop the nuclear reaction in the core of the reactor, took place within nine seconds of the tripping of the condensate pump that started the accident. The rise in the pressurizer's water level opened a relief valve that would return the pressure to normal levels.

Up to this time, the system had been automatically correcting for human errors in a satisfactory manner. The plant had been designed to correct for the loss of feedwater, a common occurrence in electric power plants, both nuclear and fossil fueled. Unfortunately, the relief valve of the pressurizer did not close once the pressure in the primary water system fell to normal values. The failure of this valve to close was complicated by a design error: instruments on the operators' control console were designed to indicate that a signal to close the valve had been sent, but not to indicate whether the valve had actually closed. On the morning of March 28, the valve remained open, a fact not known to the reactor operators. Water from the primary cooling system poured out through the open valve, causing the pressure to fall to a point where the ultimate safety system—the emergency core-cooling system—was automatically activated, feeding huge amounts of cooling water into the primary water system.

The drop in pressure in the primary cooling system led to the formation of pockets of steam, which caused the operators to conclude erroneously that the water level in the pressurizer had increased. When the operators observed this rise in water level, they reacted as they had been trained, by manually shutting down the emergency core-cooling system. Even at this point the accident could have been terminated without serious consequences.

Core meltdown would not have occurred if one last human error had not been made. About 100 minutes after the start of the accident, the continual loss of water through the open relief valve caused the two remaining cooling pumps to vibrate so violently that the operators manually shut them down. With the last possible source of cooling water removed, the water level fell below the reactor core, and 30 minutes later the core heated up to 3,500° Fahrenheit, just 280° short of the temperature required to cause the dreaded meltdown but high enough to cause severe damage to the fuel elements in the core. Four hours after the onset of the accident, more experienced supervisory personnel arrived on the scene. They realized that water was being lost through the open relief valve, which they closed, and then they restarted the emergency core-cooling system. Within 15 minutes, the reactor vessel filled with water, covering the reactor core, but it was too late. The core had been badly damaged by the combination of severe overheating and the sudden influx of cooling water.

The water pouring out of the relief valve filled a drainage tank in the reactor building. The tank then overflowed, and water containing radioactive fission products contaminated the reactor and auxiliary buildings. Two million liters of this water flooded the basement of the reactor building, reaching a depth of 2.6 meters.

Just before the Three Mile Island accident, a movie called *The China Syndrome* was being shown all over the United States. The plot centered on the dangers of nuclear power and the threat of a meltdown. During one scene, a nuclear worker said that an accident at the plant could contaminate an area "the size of Pennsylvania"; after the fact, these words gave the movie a somewhat prophetic aura.

Unlike the levels of radiation released at Chernobyl, those released at Three Mile Island were not high enough to cause radiation burns and sickness. No immediate deaths occurred, and there were no fires. Emergency medical care and triage systems were not required. The immediate response to the accident consisted of cooling the reactor, stopping damage to the core and further contamination of the containment and auxiliary fuel-handling building, and monitoring radiation levels at the plant site and throughout the surrounding community.

Within a few hours of the incident, representatives of the U.S. Nuclear Regulatory Commission and other government officials from Washington, D.C., and surrounding states arrived at the site, along with great numbers of representatives of the national and international media. Many of the statements that were released were incoherent or inaccurate. For example, groundless speculation arose that a hydrogen bubble inside the reactor was ready to explode. It took days to alleviate this fear.

Two days after the accident, the governor of Pennsylvania, Richard Thornburgh, advised all pregnant women and children within five miles of the plant to leave the area. Residents within ten miles of the plant were advised to stay indoors to reduce their exposure to radiation. William Dornsife, a nuclear engineer at the Pennsylvania Bureau of Radiation Protection and Toxicology who was involved in the response to the accident, stated: "Much later, I was to learn firsthand, from the people who were directly involved, the unfortunate series of misunderstandings that led to that Friday morning recommendation to evacuate. This event, more than anything, led to the escalation of a minor radiation release into a full-blown crisis, which continued for many days."

Ten years after the accident, the end of the cleanup process is in sight. The last of the 177 damaged fuel assemblies have been removed. It is now known that at least 70 percent of Unit 2's reactor core was damaged, and between 35 and 45 percent of its fuel assemblies were fractured during the accident. Despite the fact that 40,000 pounds of core fell to the bottom of the reactor, the reactor vessel remained intact. The reactor vessel contained a nearly 50 percent meltdown.

By 1989, when the defueling and most of the cleanup activities are scheduled to be completed, the process will have cost almost $1 billion. Removing the damaged fuel was the most difficult and expensive part. What will become of the damaged reactor has not yet been determined. Most experts agree that the reactor will never operate again. Instead, it will be put in "postdefueling monitored storage," which is analogous to putting it in mothballs. A skeletal staff will monitor the facility and its radiation levels. When Unit 2's operating twin, Unit 1, is decommissioned in the year 2010, it is likely that Unit 2 will be disassembled at the same time.

Since the accident, reactor control consoles and procedures and the qualifications and training of reactor operators all over the United States have been revised, and computer systems have been installed to aid the operators in the event of an accident. Emergency plans, including emergency response and evacuation, have been developed and tested. The experience of the accident has led to design modifications as well as a tightening of safety procedures at nuclear power plants throughout the world.

Chernobyl

In contrast to the accident at Three Mile Island, the meltdown at the nuclear power plant near the town of Chernobyl, U.S.S.R., was a technological disaster of great proportions. In some respects, the accident was comparable to major natural disasters such as earthquakes, floods, hurricanes, and volcanic eruptions, but there were also important differences. Throughout the world, fear was greatly increased because of people's unfamiliarity with radiation and radioactive materials. Moreover, the aura of secrecy that the Soviets created for thirty-six hours aggravated this fear.

Two types of power reactors are used in the Soviet Union: a pressurized-water reactor similar to those used in the Western world; and the RBMK, a graphite-moderated, boiling-water, multiple-fuel-cell reactor—the type at which the accident occurred. What led to the accident at Chernobyl was an ill-advised test to determine whether the emergency core-cooling-water pumps could be operated if the only supply of electricity was that generated by the continued rotation of the turbines after the reactor had been shut down during an emergency. To test this hypothesis, in the early morning hours of April 25, 1986, two operators sat at the control panel of the Number 4 reactor of the Chernobyl plant.

One hundred and seventy-six people were on duty at the plant, and an additional 268 construction workers constituted the night shift at the reactor site. The Number 4 reactor was the newest of four at the site, and had gone into operation in December 1983. Its basic design included 1,600 uranium dioxide fuel cells encased in zirconium alloy tubes and surrounded by graphite. In this type of reactor, the heat from nuclear reactions in the graphite-encased fuel channels converts the water into steam to drive the turbines and generate electricity. Because of the large number of fuel cells, there is no steel reactor vessel (or housing) to contain the core of the reactor as there is in most Western reactors. One characteristic of the RBMK reactor is that some of its fuel cells can be replaced while the reactor is operating. In the RBMK reactor, steam is fed directly from the fuel cells to the turbines, thereby eliminating the need for steam generators of the type found in Western reactors.

In the RBMK reactor, as in Unit 2 at Three Mile Island, six pumps control the water flowing over the 1,600 fuel channels. These pumps require electricity to operate. In the RBMK reactor, as in Western reactors, multiple sources of emergency electric power must be available at all times, and must include a supply of electricity to power the pumps; this electricity is provided by power grids outside the plant and backed up by diesel generators.

At 1:00 A.M., working under the supervision of an electrical engineer who was *not* qualified as a nuclear engineer, the reactor operators at Chernobyl slowly began to reduce the power of the reactor to try to simulate shutdown conditions. After twelve hours, the power level had been reduced from 3,200 megawatts (full power) to 1,600 megawatts. At that point, the power supply to operate the six water pumps was shifted from sources outside the plant to the turbogenerator of the Number 4 reactor itself. The reactor was thereby supplying its own emergency electricity.

The emergency core-cooling system, which had been designed to come into operation automatically if the reactor began to overheat, was intentionally deactivated by the operators, because the purpose of the test was to determine whether the reactor could generate enough electricity to activate the emergency cooling system and flood the plant with water. The power level was then further reduced as much as possible, to simulate the conditions of complete shutdown of the reactor. Under these circumstances, the reactor would continue to generate heat equivalent to about 7 percent of full power, because the radioactive fuel elements would continue to produce residual heat. At such a low power level, the reactor could not be operated by the usual automatic control systems, so the operators switched over to manual control of the position of the moderating control rods, which can stop the nuclear reaction when inserted in the proper position among the fuel cells. The operators had problems controlling the power level of the reactor and at one point the level fell to a dangerous low of 30 megawatts before it could be stabilized at 200 megawatts. All of the above events took place over an eleven-hour period.

In spite of their increasing problems, the operators did not terminate the experiment. At about 1:00 the next morning, the operators disengaged the system that would have automatically shut down the reactor in the case of overheating, because such a shutdown would have ruined the experiment. With the operators controlling the power level manually, the level continued to fall over the next fifteen minutes, eventually reaching such a low level that operating guidelines called for the reactor to be shut down immediately.

Ignoring this guideline, the operators continued to attempt to run the reactor at 200 megawatts of thermal power. When the chief operator saw that, instead, the power level was steadily and rapidly increasing, he finally decided to shut down the reactor by inserting all control and emergency rods. Because of the unusual mode in which the reactor had been operated, however, the rods were either all the way up or all the way down inside the core. The control rods did not drop low enough into the reactor to stop the nuclear reaction. Immediately (and we can only imagine his emotional state), the chief operator manually disengaged the couplings holding the rods, permitting them to drop by their own weight into the proper position. By then, it was too late. Within twenty seconds, the power increased far above its normal maximal operating level and the reactor exploded.

The explosion killed the two operators instantly. The force of the explosion blew off the roof of the reactor building and ejected burning fragments onto the roofs of adjacent buildings. Thirty fires were started, including fires in the reactor and turbine buildings. The official Soviet report of the accident stated that "the developers of the reactor installation did not envisage the creation of protective safety systems capable of preventing an accident in the presence of the set of premeditated diversions of technical protection facilities and violations of operating regulations which occurred, since they considered such a set of events impossible." Eventually, six of the people responsible for the operation of the plant at the time of the accident were tried and sentenced to from ten to twenty years at hard labor in prison camps.

As investigators later revealed, safety features that would have automatically prevented the accident—the emergency core-cooling system, for instance—had been manually disengaged. (Manual disengagement of the emergency core-cooling system was in large part responsible for the accident at Three Mile Island as well.) The operators were unbelievably reckless, had a poor understanding of the operation of a reactor, and did not appreciate the extreme danger of what they were doing.

The Soviets' response to the accident, described in the report the Soviet Union submitted to the International Atomic Energy Agency in Vienna in August 1986, was remarkably effective, except for their delay in notifying the rest of the world (especially neighboring countries) and the Soviet population of the occurrence of the accident. The first sign of the accident came in Sweden. On the morning of April 28, technicians at the Forsmark Nuclear Power Plant, sixty miles north of Stockholm, received signals that radiation levels were rising. At first, they suspected difficulties in their own reactor, but they soon found that radiation levels outside the plant were four to five times normal. The same alarming signals were being received in Norway and Denmark. Somewhere, a mysterious source was releasing radiation into the atmosphere. After the Swedes confirmed that the source was not in their country, they immediately turned their attention to their neighbor to the south, the Soviet Union. They asked Soviet officials whether an accident had occurred at Chernobyl. The Soviets initially said no, steadfastly maintaining that nothing untoward had happened.

Finally, that night, a newscaster in Moscow read these words: "An accident has taken place at the Chernobyl power station and one of the reactors was damaged. Measures are being taken to eliminate the consequences of the accident. Those affected by it are being given assistance. A government commission has been set up." This report signaled the gravest crisis that had occurred in the troubled thirty-two-year history of commercial nuclear power. Throughout the following week an anxious, puzzled, and frustrated world struggled to understand the extent of the disaster.

One hour after the explosion, twenty-nine persons were hospitalized, suffering primarily from burns. Special fire-fighting units, trained to respond to nuclear accidents, arrived from the nearby cities of Pripyat and Chernobyl. Initial efforts were directed toward preventing the fires from spreading to a nearby reactor, Number 3. Four hours after the accident, first-aid teams examined 204 fire fighters. One hundred and eight were hospitalized because of nausea and vomiting, early symptoms of acute radiation syndrome; others were sent home. Twelve hours after the accident, 3,000 physicians, 2,400 nurses, and other health professionals from around the world arrived on the scene, and within forty-eight hours they had examined 18,000 people. They prepared detailed charts and recorded laboratory data for 350 of the most seriously injured.

Robert Gale, an American physician who arrived at the scene of the accident soon after it happened, reported that the initial decision not to evacuate the population for thirty-six hours was based on the idea that taking shelter would be more effective in decreasing radiation exposure from the falling radioactive debris. Once the decision was made to act, evacuation was begun within six hours. Later, however, the Soviet government criticized local officials for delaying the evacuation of the nearby populace. Of the 135,000 people directly affected by the accident, 2 (the operators of the reactor) died from the immediate trauma of the explosion; 29 others died from a combination of thermal and radiation burns and later radiation effects. Two hundred and three persons were exposed to more than 100 rads, and 1,000,000 were exposed to more than 5 rads. The accident at Chernobyl resulted in as many deaths as occurred worldwide in nuclear accidents between 1944 and 1986: thirty-one. It also caused a state of worldwide alarm, especially in the countries surrounding the Soviet Union. This public alarm put pressure on political decision makers, and they began to take actions that were not justified on scientific grounds alone—for example, administering stable iodine to pregnant women and children in Poland.

The Aftermath

The world has not been the same since Chernobyl, just as it was not the same after the accident at Three Mile Island. As in most disasters—natural, human, or technological—the major problems at Chernobyl and Three Mile Island resulted from a lack of adequate interaction among people and institutions. In neither instance was the official response to the accident an integrated effort, but the effective medical response has made significant contributions to our understanding of such a crisis.

An important difference between the accidents at Three Mile Island and Chernobyl was that at Three Mile Island only 17 curies of radioiodine were released, because the radioactivity was kept within Unit 2's containment building. Millions of curies of the noble gases xenon-133 and krypton-85 escaped, but they rapidly diffused into the atmosphere. At Chernobyl, 50 million curies of radioactive elements, including radioiodine, were released into the atmosphere and soil over a nine-day period because of the reactor's inadequate containment and the continuous burning of large amounts of graphite in the reactor.

Today, Pripyat is a ghost town. A 30-kilometer "danger zone" surrounds the nuclear power plant. About half a million cubic meters of radioactive soil have been shaved off and buried or put in huge cement-covered vaults. Within the danger zone, 75,000 acres of land have been decontaminated and will be used again for crops. A new town at Slavutich will become the home of thousands of power plant workers and their families. At the time of this writing, most of the workers who operated the three nuclear reactors not involved in the accident live in hostels that were built after the accident on land outside the 30-kilometer danger zone.

Because of possible contamination of the reservoir supplying water to the region, 104 artesian wells were dug as soon as possible after the accident, in the vicinity of Kiev. Public use of the water from the reservoir was discontinued after the construction of the wells.

Total-body doses of radiation to people in the nearby towns of Chistowka, Levlev, Chernobyl, Rudki, and Crevichi ranged from 2 to 10 rems. Doses to the thyroids were as high as 250 rems in the town of Levlev. Cases of cancer of the thyroid and leukemia could increase by as much as 5 percent over the usual number, and this increase will be detectable if careful prospective and follow-up studies are performed. Cases of other types of cancer, however, will not be detectable over background levels.

The level of radiation to which the 45,000 people living in Pripyat were exposed was 1,560,000 person-rems, and could eventually result in 156 deaths from cancer. Because at least 9,000 of the 45,000 people will die from cancer due to all other causes, the increase resulting from the accident will not be detectable. The total number of excess cancer deaths among the 60 million people in the Soviet Union who were exposed to increased levels of radiation as a result of the accident will be approximately 2,900. Of those 60 million people, 15 million will die of cancer from all causes.

The levels of radiation to which the people around the Chernobyl power plant were exposed are in the same range as those to which the population of Hiroshima and Nagasaki were exposed in the atomic bombings of those cities in World War II. In Japan, 82,000 people who were exposed to an average dose of 27 rems of radiation have been studied carefully for decades. Of the 82,000 people studied through 1978, 91 deaths from leukemia and 160 deaths from other cancers are believed to have been caused by radiation exposure during the atomic bombings, compared to an expected cancer death rate (without the radiation exposure) of 4,500. If the Soviet population is studied with equal care for equal periods of time, the data could be of great value to scientists in determining the risk associated with various levels of exposure to radiation. Since the accident at Chernobyl, comprehensive medical surveillance of more than one million people in the Soviet Union has thus far revealed no variation from normal health patterns.

While the Soviet Union's failure to inform its citizens and surrounding nations was deplorable, the medical and technical responses to the accident were excellent. After the Three Mile Island accident, the state of preparedness of nuclear utilities, the health care systems, and the state and federal regulatory agencies in many countries were reviewed and improved. The Chernobyl accident brought about further review of emergency planning for populated areas around nuclear reactors. Experience with natural disasters has taught us that failures in emergency planning usually result from a lack of appropriate interactions among persons and institutions, rather than from deficiencies in technological or medical competence. Continual upgrading and practice of emergency procedures to integrate the response by government and private institutions and organizations is essential. Specific responses—for example, the evacuation of populations or decisions about when to administer stable iodine to exposed persons to prevent the accumulation of radioactive iodine in the thyroid glands—need to be well established and clear-cut.

In 1987, the International Commission on Radiation Protection (ICRP) recommended that a potential exposure to 5–50 rems of whole-body radiation should lead to the evacuation of a population. The commission also recommended that exposure of the thyroid glands to 0.5–5.0 rems of radiation should lead to the administration of stable iodine. These and other action levels should be reviewed in light of analogous action levels established for contaminated food. Accident alarm systems, monitoring systems, communication systems, evacuation plans, emergency planning, the setting of action levels, and education of the public need to be constantly reassessed and improved. The planned response to a nuclear accident must be international as well as national in scope. The Emergency Evacuation Planning Zones (EPZs) now required for all regions surrounding nuclear power plants in the United States, should be updated, and modified if indicated, as we obtain new knowledge and experience from accidents such as those at Three Mile Island and Chernobyl.

Two years after the accident at Chernobyl, three of the plant's four reactors are in full operation, and the fourth is entombed in concrete, emitting no radioactivity. Since the accident, five more Soviet nuclear power plants have begun operating. The construction of two additional reactors on the Chernobyl site has been canceled. Three reactors similar to the one at Chernobyl have been provided with more advanced safety systems. The plan to construct a graphite-moderated reactor of the Chernobyl type has been halted.

After the accident, A. Petrosyants, Chairman of the Soviet

State Committee on the Utilization of Atomic Energy, stated: "Nuclear power is the energy source which will have the *least damaging ecological consequences*. We feel that nuclear power will promote energy independence of individual countries and will thereby exercise a stabilizing effect on the world economy and on international relations." In November 1986 Soviet Prime Minister Nikolai I. Ryzhkov stated that by the year 2000 the U.S.S.R. and its Eastern Bloc allies intend to increase the number of nuclear power plants from fifteen to thirty-one.

Nevertheless, the Chernobyl accident was a factor in stopping the construction of a nuclear power plant near the Black Sea. According to the youth newspaper *Komsomolskaya Pravda*, the equivalent of $41 million had been spent on the Krasnodar plant before local officials bowed to a flood of letters from local residents and decided at the end of 1987 to cancel the construction of the plant. The newspaper stated in February 1988 that all of the twenty operating nuclear power plants in the country and most of those under construction were now "bitterly opposed" by local residents. Public opinion poses a serious threat to the country's ambitious nuclear energy program. According to *Komsomolskaya Pravda*, nuclear plants once lent prestige to a city, "but that was before Chernobyl." Sensitivity is particularly great in the Ukraine, where about a quarter of the country's fifty nuclear power reactors are located. Thirty Ukrainian scientists, in a letter published on January 21, 1988, in the newspaper *Literaturnaya Ukraina*, blasted on ecological grounds the government's plans to add reactors to the South Ukrainian, Khmelnitsky, and Rovno power stations. They accused the government of ignoring "the bitter lessons of Chernobyl."

The current plan is to increase the amount of electricity generated by nuclear power from 170,000 million kilowatt-hours to 360,000 million kilowatt-hours by 1990. Abandoning nuclear energy would result in an electricity shortage in the region, while the alternative to nuclear reactors—coal-fired generating plants—would bring pollution.

In the Western world, much of Europe continues to be committed to nuclear energy: nearly 70 percent of the electricity in France, 60 percent in Belgium, and 50 percent in Sweden is generated by nuclear power, but the Chernobyl accident may further delay the bringing on line of some nuclear plants presently under construction. On the other hand, although Chernobyl steeled the resolve of British environmentalists and led to extensive debate of the issue, Britain recently approved the construction of the first of a series of six new plants.

In the United States, on November 3, 1987, a referendum that would have shut down the Maine Yankee Nuclear Power plant, which supplies one-fourth of all the electricity in that state, was defeated by a vote of 59 percent to 41 percent. Previously, two similar referenda had failed to close the plant, but two new factors had entered the picture in 1987: the Chernobyl accident, and a hearing held in Maine by the U.S. Department of Energy to consider the possible establishment in Maine of a disposal site for high-level radioactive wastes. The governor and other political leaders tried to separate the two issues, but television advertisements by antinuclear groups stated that the only way to keep the disposal site out of the state would be to close the operating Maine Yankee Plant. Active opponents of the plant included the Clamshell Alliance, founded in July 1976 to oppose the construction and operation of the nuclear power plant in Seabrook, New Hampshire. That plant, conceived in the early 1970s, was delayed for years by construction problems and political and environmental opposition.

On August 1, 1976, eighteen members of the Clamshell Alliance entered the Seabrook construction site. On August 22 and 30, 1976, 180 and 2,000 persons, respectively, occupied the plant site for more than twenty-four hours. Eventually 1,415 people were arrested and imprisoned in National Guard armories for up to thirteen days. The next summer, 18 Clamshell members were arrested on the site in the first of seven "wave actions" that resulted in 107 arrests. On another occasion, 183 persons were arrested for blocking the installation of equipment in the nuclear reactor at Seabrook. Today the plant has been completed, its cost exceeding $5 billion for a single reactor. (The original plan was to produce a twin-reactor plant, at a cost of $1 billion.) The start-up of the plant has been delayed by a dispute over whether the area around the site, which is on the coast two miles north of the Massachusetts border, could be evacuated in the case of an emergency. Massachusetts officials are so opposed to the plant that they have refused to cooperate with emergency planning, which raises the strong possibility that the plant will never be licensed for full operation. In November 1987, however, the Nuclear Regulatory Commission voted to remove a key obstacle to a low-power license to test the performance of the reactor. It permitted the utility and the commission to establish an emergency plan without the involvement of Massachusetts officials. Massachusetts governor Michael Dukakis refused to have his state officials participate in the emergency evacuation plan for the nearby New Hampshire reactor.

The Future of Nuclear Energy

Despite local opposition to nuclear power plants, such as that in New England, the number of such plants worldwide is likely to continue to increase. As of September 1987, 406 operating nuclear reactors in twenty-six countries were generating 16 percent of the world's electricity. One hundred and three of these were in the United States, producing 16.6 percent of its electricity. The worldwide number is projected to increase to 496 by 1990 and to between 565 and 648 by the year 2000. These plants would increase the production of electricity by nuclear energy from approximately 250,000–394,000 megawatts in 1990 to 461,000–543,000 megawatts in 2000.

The average time from the start of construction to the start of commercial operation of the twenty-nine reactors that came into operation worldwide in 1985 was eight years. The shortest interval was recorded in Japan, where it took an average of five years to bring five new reactors into operation by 1985. The Japanese carry out all hearings, discussion, and licensing before beginning construction, after which time additional modifications are not permitted. In the United States, the construction time for the five reactors that started operating in 1985 averaged twelve years; in the U.S.S.R., the corresponding figure was eight years for four reactors; in France it was six years for three reactors; and in the Federal Republic of Germany it was eight years for three reactors. Public reaction to the Chernobyl accident may make these intervals even longer.

One useful consequence of the Chernobyl accident has been an upgrading of the International Atomic Energy Agency (IAEA), which, together with the World Health Organization, has played an important role in international activities related to the accident and is respected by most countries of the world, Eastern and Western. Among the most important functions of the IAEA is its mandate to guard against the misuse of nuclear technology to produce nuclear weapons. Eighty-seven nations have signed the Non-Proliferation Treaty, agreeing not to produce nuclear weapons, but some—Pakistan, Argentina, Brazil, India, and twenty-one other nations—have not, although they have informally agreed with the principles of the treaty.

The IAEA plays a crucial role in all aspects of the development of nuclear energy, including the management of plutonium and spent fuel, but the problem of political credibility remains. Multinational political agreements directed toward the elimination of existing nuclear weapons fall within the realm of the United Nations rather than the IAEA. Fortunately, both the United States and the Soviet Union are beginning to recognize that the nuclear arms race uses up a great deal of their nations' resources without providing anything of value in return. In the past, military strength could yield economic benefits, such as new land and markets, but this is no longer the case. Countries without the burden of huge defense spending, such as Japan, are moving ahead economically, while the two superpowers are falling steadily behind. A step in the right direction has been taken by the U.S.S.R., which has notified the IAEA that two additional Soviet nuclear facilities—the fast breeder reactor at Byeloyarsk and a spent-fuel depository at Novovoronezh—will be opened to IAEA inspection of safeguards under a "voluntary offer" agreement concluded with the agency in 1985.

Recent IAEA successes include two agreements—one on Early Notification of a Nuclear Accident, the other on Assistance in the Case of a Nuclear Accident or Radiological Emergency—both of which were stimulated by the Chernobyl accident. The Three Mile Island and Chernobyl accidents illustrate the principle that progress usually depends on problems, because the main obstacle to progress is satisfaction with the status quo.

According to Richard Wilson, Mallinckrodt Professor of Physics at Harvard University and an expert on nuclear reactor safety,

> the commitment of the Soviet Union to nuclear power is in stark contrast to the implicit and often blatant calls for abandoning nuclear power in the United States. . . . To take the

path of abandoning a technology because of one accident would put a nation on a backward trend. . . . This is symptomatic of a broader dissatisfaction with and misunderstanding of modern technology. Economic progress requires that we move forward with industrial technologies, while pragmatically learning to master the important principles of accident prevention, management and recovery. The nation that applies these technologies will lead the world. If the United States shrinks from the challenge in the false belief that it cannot control technologies, such as nuclear power, Nikita Khrushchev's famous prediction—that the Soviets will bury us—may yet come to pass.

NUCLEAR WASTE DISPOSAL: NOT IN MY BACKYARD

Six-year-old Leide Das Neves Ferreira, the niece of a Brazilian scrap metal dealer, died on October 23, 1987, several days after rubbing cesium-137 on her hands and then eating a hard-boiled egg. Her 37-year-old aunt, Maria Gabriela Ferreira, died on the same day, also from overexposure to radiation. The scrap metal dealer had removed a 500-pound radiation therapy device from an abandoned radiation center, a clinic in the town of Goiania, Brazil, and brought it home.

To salvage the steel container, Mr. Alves used a sledge hammer to remove the protective covering around the radiation source, and found "something like a blue crystal." What he found was a deadly amount of the radioactive substance cesium-137. Believing that the glowing object might have magical powers, the Alves family kept it in their home, proudly displaying it to relatives and friends. They rubbed the colored material over their bodies and carried small pieces around in their pockets. Leide's father, Ivo Ferreira, scraped some powder off with a screwdriver, brought it to his house, and sprinkled it on the floor of the children's room, where he said it "gave light, like a firefly."

A few days later, several townspeople began to experience nausea, vomiting, second-degree radiation burns, generalized aches and pains, and gastrointestinal bleeding—symptoms of acute radiation syndrome. By the time public health officials realized what had happened, 44 people had been hospitalized with serious contamination and 245 others were believed to have been exposed to some level of radiation. Some townspeople panicked and fled the town of Goiania, while 34,000 others stood in lines at the soccer stadium to be examined with radiation detectors. Those who were found to have significant amounts of radioactivity on their bodies were instructed to take five daily showers with detergents and vinegar, to rub a "cleansing paste" on their skin, and to take medicine to help expel the cesium-137 from their bodies. President José Sarney Costa ordered police surveillance and identification checks at Brazil's main airports to try to intercept those who were believed responsible for abandoning the cesium-filled device.

This tragedy painfully illustrates what can happen if high-level radioactive waste is not properly disposed of by persons who are trained to handle it. There are safe ways to dispose of radioactive waste. The lack of effective disposal systems for high- and low-level radioactive wastes is the result of political rather than scientific or technological problems. The mere thought of a nuclear waste facility in a community often causes fear and panic, and can spell the end of the careers of politicians who favor such a facility. A "not in my backyard" mentality is the major obstacle to the safe disposal of radioactive wastes. *Political* solutions have not yet been found, and will require considerable education of the public as to the risks of radiation, both real and perceived.

The public accepts the risks of radioactive smoke alarms, the use of radiation to sterilize nipples for baby bottles, sterilized hospital supplies, coated paper for magazines and books, luminous dials, emergency exit signs, just to name a few of the uses of ionizing radiation in daily life. The electricity we take for granted in the United States, nearly 17 percent of which is generated by 106 nuclear power plants, would no longer be available if we prohibited further production of radioactive wastes. Most biomedical research would grind to a halt and pharmaceutical companies could not test new drugs for safety and effectiveness if there were no way to dispose of radioactive wastes. More than 95 percent of all prescription drugs that have been approved by the U.S. Food and Drug Administration were initially tested with radioactive tracers.

In 1985, in an official letter sent to Senator Strom Thurmond of South Carolina and Congressman Morris K. Udall of Arizona, the American Medical Association stated that "the development of low-level waste disposal facilities and sites is important to protect public health." Because our health care system depends on radioactive materials, the answer lies not in preventing the production of all radioactive wastes but in developing the proper methods for their disposal.

There are two types of radioactive waste, "low level" and "high level." In general, low-level waste is defined as that which contains low concentrations of radioactivity in a large volume of material. High-level waste has radioactivity highly concentrated in a small volume of material. Radioactive waste is also classified according to the amount of radioactivity present and the half-lives of the radionuclides involved.

The Low-Level Radioactive Waste Policy Act of 1980 divided low-level waste into three classes. Class A waste, which has a low concentration of radionuclides, covers the vast majority of low-level waste (examples include trash, paper, plastics, low-specific-activity resins, animal carcasses, and other wastes from medical and/or research institutions). Class B waste has a moderate concentration of radionuclides with short half-lives and a low concentration of radionuclides with long half-lives (examples include evaporator concentrates, resins, and filters from nuclear power plants and medical radionuclide production facilities). Class C waste has high concentrations of short-lived and/or long-lived radionuclides (examples include some of the waste from power plants).

The Nuclear Waste Policy Act of 1982 defined high-level waste as spent fuel from nuclear power plants, transuranic waste, mill tailings, and highly radioactive waste. The uranium pellets that power nuclear reactors are encapsulated in long, cylindrical zirconium-metal canisters called "fuel rods," which need to replaced about every three years because the waste material that accumulates within the rods impedes the efficiency of the fission process. "Transuranic elements," also called "actinides," are elements that are heavier than uranium, which has an atomic number of 92. Plutonium, einsteinium, fermium, and nobelium are transuranics. Mill tailings, a by-product of the mining and processing of uranium, consist of large quantities of naturally radioactive rock and soil containing radium, which decays into radon gas. Highly radioactive waste is a self-boiling, intensely radioactive liquid that results from the separation of fission products, such as strontium and cesium, and transuranics, from uranium and plutonium during the reprocessing of spent nuclear fuel rods.

In the United States, more than 20,000 civilian companies and institutions, including more than 3,300 medical facilities, routinely use radioactive materials and generate low-level waste. Low-level radioactive waste makes up an exceedingly small fraction—about 0.007 percent—of the total weight of all solid waste produced annually in the United States. Types of solid waste include: agricultural (3 billion tons per year), mining and milling (2.3 billion tons per year), industrial (400 million tons), municipal (200 million tons), utility ash and sludge (100 million tons), and low-level radioactive waste (40,000 tons). Low-level waste makes up 2 percent of the volume and 1 percent of the radioactivity of all civilian nuclear waste.

Since the 1940s, when the nuclear era began in the United States, two methods of disposal of low-level waste have been used: ocean dumping and shallow land burial. Years ago, the Atomic Energy Commission dumped contaminated glassware, animal carcasses, and other laboratory items into the Atlantic and Pacific oceans. In 1960, the commission declared a moratorium on issuing new ocean disposal licenses, and began opening up land burial sites, including the facilities at Oak Ridge, Tennessee, and Idaho Falls, Idaho. Land burial was less expensive than ocean dumping, and by 1962, about 95 percent of all low-level waste in the United States was stored in land burial sites. In 1970, the United States ceased dumping radioactive waste into the ocean.

Despite considerable public protest, sea disposal of low-level radioactive waste is still an officially accepted practice in some Western European countries. At times, members of the organization Greenpeace have physically attempted to prevent the disposal of radioactive waste in the ocean. According to the International Atomic Energy Agency in Vienna, however, the amount of radioactivity deposited in the ocean is very small compared to the natural radioactivity already present in those waters and has not measurably increased the radioactivity levels of the ocean.

National laboratories in the United States, formerly funded by the Atomic Energy Commission (AEC) and now funded by the U.S. Department of Energy (DOE), developed their own shallow land burial facilities and initially accepted radioactive waste from private companies and medical/research facilities. By 1960, however, in typical American fashion, the fast growth in commercial uses of radioactive materials had prompted the AEC to propose that the private sector develop commercial disposal sites for its low-level waste.

The first commercial disposal site opened in 1962 in Beatty, Nevada. Later that year, the Maxey Flats disposal site, in eastern Kentucky, became available. In 1963 the West Valley disposal site, in western New York, began operation. Another site opened in 1964 at the Hanford Reservation, near Richland, Washington, and in 1967 a disposal site was established in Sheffield, Illinois. The sixth and most recently built commercial radioactive-waste facility in the United States, at Barnwell, South Carolina, entered the disposal business in 1971.

Several government facilities have encountered problems in the disposal of radioactive waste. The DOE facility in Fernald, Ohio, which processes uranium for nuclear weapons, has been cited for inadequate monitoring of groundwater, incomplete analyses of wastes, and incomplete plans for closure of the facility. Inadequate groundwater monitoring has also been charged at the Portsmouth, Ohio, Uranium Enrichment Plant, which produces enriched uranium reactor fuel. The Savannah River Plant, in Aiken, South Carolina, which produces plutonium and tritium for thermonuclear weapons, and the Hanford facility, in Richland, Washington, have been cited for inadequate groundwater monitoring and for releasing hazardous materials, including trichloroethane, into the groundwater and soil.

In fact, groundwater penetration of some storage trenches forced officials to close three disposal sites—West Valley in 1975, Maxey Flats in 1977, and Sheffield in 1978. That left only three sites to handle the nation's growing volume of low-level radioactive waste. Despite the enormous economic benefits that accrued to their states from operating the sites, the governors of Nevada, Washington, and South Carolina let it be known that their states would not indefinitely shoulder the entire burden of this country's disposal of low-level waste.

As a result of the near monopoly created by these three disposal sites, the cost of waste storage increased to the point where the disposal costs almost matched the cost of the original radioactive materials before use. Nevertheless, the managers of the Beatty and Richland sites became so frustrated by customers who were careless about following transportation and packaging regulations that they temporarily shut down those two facilities in 1979. The Barnwell site remained open, but the governor of South Carolina ordered a phased monthly reduction in the volume of waste accepted. Congress responded to the disposal crisis by passing the Low-Level Radioactive Waste Policy Act of 1980, which made each state responsible for its own low-level waste and encouraged states to establish regional disposal sites. Complex negotiations among states, as well as assessments of potential disposal sites for low-level waste, are still going on today, while the costs of storing radioactive waste continue to soar.

In 1983, the U.S. Nuclear Regulatory Commission (NRC) promulgated comprehensive regulations governing commercial land disposal of low-level radioactive waste. The regulations require that no individual be exposed to more than 25 millirems per year (about one-quarter of the total received from natural background radiation) from a disposal site. To meet this objective, planners of disposal sites for low-level waste need to consider many factors, including geology, hydrology, seismology, natural resources, population density, and nearby activities.

Public hearings must be held before the NRC will grant a license. Disposal-site operators must devise a plan for closing the facility when it is full, and sufficient funds for monitoring and maintenance must be assured for up to 100 years. Trenches for shallow land burial are typically 600 feet long, 100 feet wide, and 25 feet deep. The contents of each shipment are recorded and the containers are placed methodically within the trenches. Class A waste requires "safe handling and packaging," whereas Class B and Class C waste must be stored so that it retains its size and shape for 300 years. Class C waste must be buried deeper than Class A and Class B waste, and must be protected from intrusion for 500 years. Some states are looking at alternatives to shallow land burial, such as above-ground vaults, underground cells, and earth-mounded concrete bunkers.

Incineration is another method commonly used to dispose of low-level radioactive waste. Research facilities and manufacturing firms that have permits to carry out on-site incineration avoid the expense and problems associated with transporting this waste to another location. An uninformed public, however, can engender fear and panic—and even hysteria—when a local institution expresses its intention to incinerate radioactive waste.

For example, during a meeting in New York City on November 16, 1983, the City Council's Committee on Environmental Protection held a hearing to decide whether low-level radioactive and chemical waste from Rockefeller University could be incinerated. Rosalyn S. Yalow, the nuclear physicist who received the Nobel Prize in Physiology or Medicine in 1977, gave the following testimony in support of the proposal:

> Rockefeller University for two years has requested permission to incinerate annually, under carefully controlled conditions, one-tenth of a Curie of tritium and five-thousandths of a Curie of carbon-14. This is less than one-thousandth the natural carbon-14 burned in the city garbage and less than one-hundredth the natural tritium in the city rainfall each year. . . . If one were to ban release into the air of any radioactive material in New York City, it would be necessary to close down all municipal garbage incinerators and landfills since the city's garbage releases 20 Curies of carbon-14 into the air annually. All coal-burning power plants and heating units in the city would have to be banned as well because they release natural radioactivity from the radium family into the atmosphere. In fact, at 100 feet from the Rockefeller incinerator stack, inhaling the radioactive emission due to the effluent they have requested to burn would result in less radiation exposure to the lining of the human lungs than cooking with natural gas, which has self-contained natural radioactivity. Are we also to ban cooking and heating with natural gas in the city?

Yalow is an outspoken scientist who has been called "Madame Curie of the Bronx." She was awarded the Nobel Prize for her work with the late Solomon Berson, of the Bronx Veterans Administration Medical Center, in developing the radioimmunoassay, a technique that revolutionized science and medicine by giving physicians and scientists an exquisitely sensitive and specific tool for measuring minute quantities of many substances, such as insulin, in the blood and other body fluids. During the 1983 hearing on incineration, she strongly criticized Manhattan's borough president for comparing the burning of radioactive waste from medical research with the problems at Love Canal and Three Mile Island. She also criticized New York City's commissioner of health and other officials who testified that the incineration was dangerous.

Yalow was scolded for attacking and insulting city officials, and accused of being "a paid representative of Rockefeller University." As a scientist dedicated to pursuing nuclear medical research for almost forty years, Yalow resented the accusation, noting that she had always taken time out from her research to lend her expertise to government bodies that were trying to formulate standards and regulations for the safe use of radioactive materials. She pointed out that she had testified numerous times at hearings of congressional committees, the NRC, and other organizations—never as a paid representative of any party with a vested interest, but always as a scientist fighting against the illogical imposition of unnecessarily strict radiation safety regulations that impede medical research. In the spirit of the "original Madame Curie," she had declined offers to serve as a consultant to companies that manufacture radioimmunoassay kits "because then I would not be free to speak my mind."

Rockefeller University's proposed release of radioactive materials into the environment of New York City posed no health hazards. Despite the fact that residents of Denver, Colorado, are exposed to twice as much background radiation as residents of New York City, the incidence of cancer is lower in Denver than in New York City, which indicates that factors other than low-level radiation are involved in causing cancer. At the November 16 hearing, Edward Gershey, of Rockefeller University, pointed out: "One of the serious consequences of a negative ruling in this case by the Board of Health would be setting unrealistically low levels for permissible exposure to radioactivity for the people in the City of New York. The implications would be that one would logically have to ban eating cereals, riding subways, visiting Grand Central Station or city skyscrapers, and other activities that expose persons to the same amount of radiation as would be released from the incinerator."

In 1983, the U.S. Environmental Protection Agency (EPA) proposed a maximum exposure of 10 millirems per year to any organ of an individual living near a medical facility that discharges radioactive material into the air. The president of The Society of Nuclear Medicine testified before the EPA against such a regulation, pointing out that the variations in background radiation levels throughout the country are much greater than 10 millirems per year, yet no increased incidence of cancer is found in regions, such as Colorado, where the public is exposed to much higher doses of radiation. He further noted that the nation's medical facilities already comply with the NRC regulations that set limits on the yearly discharge of various radionuclides into the air and water. The EPA eventually decided not to try to control airborne radioactive emissions, explaining that "the total risk from radionuclide emissions to air from all NRC-licensed facilities and non-DOE federal facilities is no more than 0.001 fatal cancer cases per year, or one case in every 1,000 years. The risk to nearby individuals exposed to the most concentrated of the plants' emissions is about two in 100,000." (The chances of an individual's developing cancer without this added radiation exposure are one in four.) The Sierra Club filed suit against the EPA (*Sierra Club v. Ruckelshaus*), however, forcing the agency once again to try to establish standards.

The biological and medical research communities felt squeezed as the number of disposal sites for low-level radioactive waste decreased and the sites that remained increased their prices. Reducing the volume of radioactive waste became a top priority for hospitals, universities, research laboratories, and radiopharmaceutical companies. As the radiation safety officer from the National Institutes of Health (NIH) explained, a researcher may start out with a very small volume, such as one milliliter, of radioactive material in a highly concentrated form. Throughout the course of an experiment, however, a much greater volume of radioactive waste is produced, including bench paper, paper towels and tissues, rubber gloves, beakers and other glassware, plastic items, syringes, laboratory coats and other protective clothing, liquids, biological specimens, cell cultures, animal carcasses, and animal and human excreta.

All radioactive waste at the NIH and other large biomedical institutions is brought to a central area for processing, where it is sorted, segregated, assayed, monitored, solidified, and packaged for incineration, storage, or transport to a disposal site for low-level waste. Animal carcasses that are contaminated with radiation at a level too high for incineration, according to NRC regulations, are stored in a large freezer until the radioactivity decays to an acceptable level for incineration. At the NIH, liquid waste is stored in two 10,000-gallon underground tanks until the radioactivity has decayed to a level low enough for dumping into the sanitary sewage system.

Liquid scintillation counting, an analytical technique used in research laboratories, produces a unique class of low-level radioactive waste consisting of small glass or plastic vials that usually contain 5–10 milliliters of fluid. This fluid is a mixture of chemicals known as a "scintillation cocktail," an experimental sample that is analyzed by measuring its radioactivity. The vials usually also contain toluene or xylene, which means that they must be managed as radioactive *and* chemical waste.

Biomedical institutions account for 55 percent of the volume of all low-level radioactive waste in the United States but only 3 percent of the radioactivity. Liquid scintillation vials account for 40 percent of the volume of low-level waste, yet they make up only 0.1 percent of the radioactivity. The need to reduce the volume of low-level waste has focused attention on an important concept in radiation safety and government regulations: *de minimis*, or concentrations "below regulatory concern." *De minimis*, a Latin phrase meaning "the least," is used to describe quantities of potential pollutants that are too minute to cause measurable harm to the environment.

In November 1979, Rosalyn Yalow explained to a congressional committee why the federal government needs to establish *de minimis* levels for radioactive waste:

> As a living adult human being, my body contains natural radioactivity, 0.1 microcurie of potassium-40 and 0.1 microcurie of carbon-14. According to the current rules of the NRC, if I were a laboratory animal who had received this amount of radioactivity as a "by-product material" and died with the radioactivity still within my body, I could not be buried, burned, or otherwise disposed of. I would have to be placed in a drum and transported to a low-level radioactive waste disposal site, thereafter to needlessly occupy space that should be reserved for measurably hazardous material.

The NRC reacted quickly and in March 1981 published new

rules permitting scintillation fluids and animal carcasses containing less than 0.05 microcurie of tritium (hydrogen-3) or carbon-14 per gram to be disposed of as nonradioactive waste. This NRC rule went into effect before the U.S. Department of Transportation made the same change in its rules on transporting hazardous waste. For a time, these scintillation vials and animal carcasses still had to be labeled as radioactive materials during transport to a disposal facility, but once there, they were classified as nonradioactive material, thereby causing much confusion for disposal-site operators.

In an address to the American Chemical Society in 1986, Rosalyn Yalow said that much more needs to be done to reduce the volume of low-level radioactive waste. The annual cost for packing materials, transport, and disposal of biomedical low-level waste was about $20 million in 1979, and that cost doubled over the next five years. In 1988, it cost between $100 and $400 to ship one fifty-five-gallon drum of low-level radioactive waste from New York City to Richland, Washington, and some of the shipments containing iodine-125 (half-life = 60 days) or phosphorus-32 (half-life = 14 days) were not even radioactive by the time they arrived.

The disposal of high-level radioactive waste presents an even greater challenge than that of low-level waste, although much smaller volumes are involved. To keep a nuclear power reactor operating efficiently in the production of electricity, 25–35 percent (about 30 tons) of the reactor's fuel rods must be replaced each year. These contain about 29 tons of the original uranium, 0.8 tons of fission products (including 0.23 tons of plutonium), and 0.2 tons of transuranic elements. Spent fuel rods from reactors that produce nuclear weapons are reprocessed to recover the usable uranium and plutonium. During his term of office, President Jimmy Carter prohibited the reprocessing of spent fuel rods from commercial nuclear reactors in the United States, in an attempt to restrict the diversion of plutonium to the production of nuclear weapons. President Ronald Reagan lifted that ban in 1981, but required that private industry rather than the government provide funding for nuclear-fuel-reprocessing plants. Since the growth of nuclear energy in the United States has slowed to almost a standstill, no private companies have risked investing in such reprocessing plants. Furthermore, there has been concern that shipments of plutonium and enriched uranium from existing or future reprocessing plants in Europe and Japan might reach the hands of terrorists. Although the DOE, the State Department, the Arms Control and Disarmament Agency, and the NRC all agree with the standards set by the International Atomic Energy Agency to prevent the diversion of civilian uranium or plutonium to military use, the Department of Defense has claimed that the security of these shipments is not strict enough. According to the Pentagon, as many as three hundred shipments (containing more than 25,000 kilograms of plutonium) leave European reprocessing plants annually, and if terrorists succeeded in capturing even a small amount (perhaps 10 kilograms) of processed plutonium, they could feasibly build a crude nuclear bomb.

The volume of liquid radioactive waste produced each year by a 1,000-megawatt nuclear power plant is twenty cubic meters. This material is initially stored in specially designed stainless steel dual-wall tanks that are continuously cooled. After about ten years, the radioactivity of the material decreases to a point where long-term storage becomes possible. The waste is then converted into glass and stored for ten to fifteen years in wells. The volume of this vitrified radioactive waste is about two cubic meters rather than twenty.

Several alternative methods of storage after vitrification have been proposed and are at varying stages of development and evaluation. Most of these methods involve solidifying high-level radioactive waste in borosilicate glass. The glass blocks would then be encased in stainless steel, enclosed in a succession of interacting multiple barriers made of lead, titanium, cast iron, reinforced concrete, and asphalt—like the layers of an onion—and finally immobilized underground. For about fifty years the canisters would be monitored and the waste would be retrievable, but then the storage chambers would be filled with crushed rock.

The basic premise of this method is that strong glass and stable geologic formations can safely contain high-level radioactive waste for thousands if not millions of years. This is not as far-fetched as it may sound. Unbroken glass artifacts from ancient civilizations that flourished 3,500 years ago are on exhibit today in museums such as the Corning Glass Museum in upstate New York. Fossilized insects millions of years old have been found preserved in amber. Mammoths buried in glaciers 30,000 years ago have been found with fresh meat still on their bones. The Egyptian pyramids isolated many objects, providing a relatively permanent barrier between them and the outside environment. Some scientists point out that the earth has already demonstrated its ability to contain high-level radioactive waste for millions of years. About 1.8 billion years ago, a uranium deposit saturated with water near what is now Oklo, Gabon, in East Africa, formed a critical mass, resulting in a fission chain reaction. This prehistoric natural reactor operated for more than 100,000 years, producing ten tons of high-level nuclear waste. Over the course of millions of years, most of the solid fission products, and essentially all of the transuranic elements, remained locked within the deposit and decayed until they were no longer radioactive.

Current plans in the United States call for the disposal of high-level radioactive waste in geologic repositories—vaults carved out of solid rock at least 1,000 feet below the earth's surface. All types of high-level waste except uranium mill tailings (which are now stored in large outdoor sand piles in Colorado, New Mexico, South Dakota, Texas, Utah, Washington, and Wyoming) will eventually be stored in the underground vaults or tombs of such repositories. Tourists and pilgrims who have visited the Valley of the Fallen, a shrine and mausoleum of Franco about sixty kilometers from Madrid, Spain, have seen an analogous engineering feat. Built during the 1940s and 1950s, the religious monument comprises a hospice, monastery, study center, esplanade, massive sculptures of saints, a 150-meter-high stone cross, and a basilica or crypt. With the exception of the underground crypt, these structures rise out of an isolated, cone-shaped crag of bare rock in a remote valley of the Sierra de Guadarrama. The crypt, 262 meters long and 41 meters high, was carved out of solid rock.

How long must high-level radioactive waste be contained and isolated? The EPA has stipulated that geologic repositories be built so that the radionuclides stay within 10 kilometers of the burial site for at least 10,000 years. The National Academy of Sciences' National Research Council has recommended that the long-term probable release should be low enough that no individual would be exposed to more than 10 percent of natural background radiation.

Others have proposed that the high-level waste must be contained until its radioactivity has decayed to the same level as natural uranium ore deposits—which for the high-level liquid waste produced when fuel rods are reprocessed would take approximately 500–20,000 years, and for unreprocessed spent fuel rods, 3 million years. It has been calculated that it would take several hundred thousand years for geologic faults and/or groundwater to erode the multiple layers of intentionally constructed barriers and allow the nuclear waste to escape into the environment.

A key question is how to warn future generations to stay away from the entombed high-level waste. A universal type of communication could become necessary thousands of years from now if records are lost or destroyed and civilizations and languages fade away, to be replaced by new ones. Some people have likened nuclear facilities and disposal sites for high-level radioactive waste to religious shrines, monitored perpetually by an "atomic priesthood" of scholars and scientists that would appoint new members as older ones passed away. An anthropologist has suggested adopting techniques from ancient civilizations that kept generations of people away from certain forbidden sites—the tomb of King Tut, for example. Redundant messages could be inscribed at the site in three ways: iconically (in a pictorial sequence), indexically (in a physical demonstration), and symbolically (through language). Every 100 years, the information could be updated and rewritten in the current language.

While storage of radioactive waste does not present a technical problem, the political problems of selecting storage sites are immense. The U.S. Department of Energy (DOE) has narrowed the possible location of the nation's first permanent repository for high-level waste to: the Hanford facility in Richland, Washington (which has a deposit of basalt rock of volcanic origin); Nye County, Nevada (in which there is a deposit of tuff rock of volcanic origin); and Deaf Smith and Swishers counties, in the Texas panhandle (where bedded salt formations are found).

As exemplified by a recent conflict between the DOE and Congress, the disposal of high-level radioactive waste is a political—not a technological—problem. During the summer of 1987, Congressman Morris K. Udall of Arizona introduced a bill that would take away DOE's authority to oversee the civilian high-level radioactive waste program because DOE had abandoned the original plans for selecting a second geologic repository, possibly in the Eastern United States. Western states have expressed resentment at being placed high on the list for geologic repositories when most of the nuclear waste is being generated in the Eastern states.

According to a report in *Radwaste News*, a bimonthly newsletter,

> most senators, representatives, governors, and state legislators are supportive of DOE's decision. . . . The most influential of [the statesmen who structured the Nuclear Waste Policy Act of 1982] is . . . Morris Udall of Arizona who single-handedly pushed the bill through the House and, literally in the last minutes of the Congressional session, it passed the Senate. . . . Udall had some harsh words for DOE. "Nuclear waste can be disposed of safely, but the site must be chosen carefully and on the basis of geology," said Udall. "We do our constituents no service by blocking the siting of a permanent geologic repository. Almost all of us already have a de facto nuclear waste dump closer to home than we care to think. . . . The DOE had an unpopular and thankless task in selecting the sites, to be sure, but it had only to follow faithfully the process we laid down. The fact is, . . . DOE blew it. At the first sign of public opposition, they cast aside the entire second repository program to help a few office seekers. . . . It seems to me that a large part of our trouble with this issue stems from the public perception of nuclear waste repositories as a source of endless misfortune. We need to turn this perception around. We need to assure the public of the safety of any repository, and to make hosting a repository attractive through jobs, federal grants, road improvements, land transfers—whatever the host state may reasonably request."

This incentive approach may, in fact, reverse the public's negative perception. Nevada politicians, for example, have generally been opposed to a high-level waste disposal site in their state. Recently, however, one office holder reportedly implied that if "the pie were sweetened" by Congress's choosing Nevada as the site for the superconducting supercollider (a high-energy physics research facility), opposition to the high-level waste site could diminish. The Nuclear Waste Policy Act of 1982 stipulates that Indian tribes, as well as states, can reject a geologic repository in their jurisdictions and that both houses of Congress must vote to override those decisions.

In addition to worrying about the potential risks of burying high-level nuclear waste, many people worry about the safety of transporting the waste to the disposal site. Among the general public, there is a widely held misconception that methods of reducing risk during transportation have not yet been developed. Many people mistakenly believe that no spent fuel rods have ever been transported along public thoroughfares in the United States. In actuality, since 1973 more than 800 shipments (containing more than 1,000 spent fuel rod assemblies) have been made by truck, and more than 100 shipments (about 1,000 assemblies) have been made by railroad. In durability tests, the casks that carry spent fuel rods during transport have been rammed into concrete walls at eighty miles per hour, dropped from heights of thirty feet, and exposed to 1,475° Fahrenheit fires for up to thirty minutes without breaking their seals. Despite all of these precautions, however, no one can ever *guarantee* that a leak will not occur during a traffic accident or train crash—just as no one can ever guarantee that life-threatening accidents and exposures to potential carcinogens will not happen during other activities that we pursue.

Several countries—including Belgium, Canada, Czechoslovakia, Finland, France, West Germany, India, Italy, Japan, the Netherlands, the Soviet Union, Sweden, Switzerland, and the United Kingdom—are pursuing their own solutions for disposing of high-level nuclear waste. Some of these countries export their spent fuel to other countries for reprocessing. Almost all of these countries, however, have established plans to solidify the high-level waste in glass, encase the glass in multiple layers, and bury it in stable geologic repositories.

Some scientists believe that the best method of disposing of nuclear waste would be to bury it far beneath the ocean floor, as far away as possible from areas inhabited by human beings. These scientists realize, however, that the international politics involved in such a project would be quite complicated. Nevertheless, the dean of the Woods Hole Oceanographic Institute, in Massachusetts, has pointed out that the clays in the central ocean basins have been geologically stable for more than 100 million years. These clays also have the highest ion-exchange coefficient of any geologic body, which means that radioactivity would bind more tightly to this clay than to the types of rock found in other proposed repositories. High-level waste could be buried 100 feet below the ocean floor for about the same cost as land-based disposal, according to some estimates. Here, as in most other issues involving radioactive waste, political concerns and an exaggerated perception of risk play important roles. As Morris Udall has pointed out, nuclear waste is now being stored in temporary facilities throughout the United States and other countries. In the ongoing debate, the effects of misinformation are doing far more damage, are costing more, and are wasting more resources than any other factor.

RADON BECOMES A HOUSEHOLD WORD

Radon became a hot news item on August 14, 1986, when the U.S. Environmental Protection Agency (EPA) announced at a press conference: "Radon is the biggest public health problem that radiation experts have acknowledged for years." On this day, the EPA announced that radon may cause 5,000–20,000 of the 130,000 total lung cancer deaths that occur in the United States each year. The EPA also set an "action level" of 4 pCi/l, meaning that it recommends that homeowners who find 4 picocuries (10^{-12} or 1/1,000,000,000,000 of a curie) or more of radioactivity per liter of air in their houses should take some action to determine whether a significant health hazard exists. Four picocuries per liter represents the decay of eight radon atoms per minute in a liter of air.

What exactly is radon? Radon is a radioactive gas produced when uranium decays. Uranium and its decay products (also called "daughters") are everywhere on earth, although radon concentrations vary from place to place. All soils and rocks contain at least traces of radon. In some regions, the concentrations are high. If you extracted the top foot of soil from an average square mile of earth—about 1.7 million tons of soil—you would find about three tons of uranium, six tons of thorium, and one gram of radium. All three of these elements produce radioactive gases—radon and thoron—that continually escape from the ground and account for the major portion of natural environmental radiation.

Since uranium is so widely distributed throughout the earth, miners are exposed to more radon than workers in other occupations. In general, this holds true for uranium, fluorspar, zinc, lead, and iron miners. Coal and uranium deposits, however, are not usually found together, so coal miners are not exposed to unusual amounts of radon. Black shales, phosphate rock, granites, and carbonate rocks contain higher-than-average concentrations of uranium. The Reading Prong, for example, is a mass of black shale that runs parallel to the Appalachian Mountains, beginning near Reading, Pennsylvania, and extending northeast to Trenton, New Jersey. This geologic formation played a pivotal role in raising public awareness of radon—transforming it from a mining problem to a potential problem for every household.

On December 19, 1984, when Stanley J. Watras arrived at work, he set off radiation detector alarms at the Limerick Nuclear Power Station in Pennsylvania. Radon daughter products were found in his hair and clothes, and were eventually traced back to his household air. Tests revealed a count of 2,700 pCi/l in his Colebrookdale Township house—the highest environmental level of radon ever recorded, and 675 times higher than the recommended EPA level. Watras, the father of three very young children, moved his family to another house, quit smoking cigarettes, and began a crusade for more epidemiological research on the health effects of radon exposure.

The major potential risk posed by radon comes from inhaling its daughter products, polonium-218 and polonium-214, which emit alpha radiation. Unlike radon, a noble gas, radon daughters are chemically active; they combine readily with other chemicals and adhere to the bronchial mucosa of the lungs, potentially causing lung cancer. Alpha radiation consists of positively charged subatomic particles (containing two protons and two neutrons) emitted from the nucleus of certain radioactive atoms. This type of radiation is much less penetrating than gamma rays or X-rays, and a piece of thin paper or the human skin can stop it. Mucus in the lungs can help prevent alpha particles from reaching lung tissue. While the energy from gamma rays and X-rays is absorbed over a larger area of body tissue, that from alpha particles is highly concentrated on a much smaller amount of tissue, and therefore has the potential to cause more local damage.

Watras remains a strong advocate of nuclear power. "The radiation exposure I received in 12 years as a nuclear worker was 1,000–2,000 times less than the exposures received by my family in the one year we lived in our house," he initially pointed out. After consulting with numerous physicians about the health effects their family might suffer from living with so much radon, however, the Watrases became more and more uncertain: "We repeatedly heard 'I don't know' from doctors when we asked about the health risks, and that was truly emotionally damaging for me and my wife. When we tried to find the answer, we came up with the same thing everyone else comes up with—mathematical speculations."

Most of the data used in estimating the risk of radon in the home come from studies of miners. Health effects occurring at high radiation exposures are used to estimate what might happen at low doses, the same approach that is used in other estimates of the risk of low-level radiation exposure. As early as the sixteenth century, silver miners in Joachimsthal (in what is now Czechoslovakia) were dying of an unknown lung disease. The mysterious disease remained unknown until 1889, when two mine physicians recognized that these men were dying of lung cancer. Their lesions usually formed down to the level of about six branchings of the upper airways but never deep within the lungs, which suggested that something being inhaled might be causing the cancer. The level of radon and its decay products in these mines with high uranium deposits was approximately 500 pCi/l. (U.S. houses, by comparison, contain an average of 1 pCi/l of radon, resulting in an estimated annual exposure of 1.5 rems to the bronchial epithelium.)

In studies of 3,000 American miners who retired in the early 1970s and whose bronchial epithelium had been exposed to 40 rems per year for an average of ten years, lung cancer was found in 250 miners. None of them developed the disease before the age of forty, and the *minimum* interval between exposure and the development of lung cancer was five years; smoking greatly increased the risk. By extrapolating these data to lower radon levels found in homes, epidemiologists calculate that the risk of lung cancer from radon in an average home ranges between 1 in 100 and 1 in 500, or that 0.2–1.0 percent of all people living in these houses will die of radon-caused lung cancer. According to these calculations, when a non-smoker dies of lung cancer, the chances are 20–50 percent that radon caused the disease; when a smoker dies of lung cancer, the chances are 5–10 percent that radon caused it.

Research is still continuing. It is important to remember that many factors determine whether a person will develop cancer. In Maine, for example, scientists are studying the effects of radon in well water. (The major risk from radon in water comes not from drinking or bathing but from the radon released into household air from running water, particularly showers.) In addition to measuring radon in homes, the Maine researchers asked homeowners questions about active and passive smoking history, occupational exposures, medical histories, and household characteristics. It's also important to look at the *type* of lung cancer that develops. For example, there is very little evidence that adenocarcinomas are induced by radon, yet almost half of all lung cancers in nonsmoking women are adenocarcinomas. As Stanley Watras said, "It's possible that exposure to radon is not as dangerous as it is perceived today. Perhaps the data will show that it's actually beneficial. But until some more thorough, prospective epidemiologic studies are completed, we have to assume the worst and hope for the best."

The radon issue is another example of the importance of distinguishing between real and perceived risks. Although we are still learning about the "real" risks, it is possible to find reasonable estimates and compare them with other risks of life. By learning how radon exposure compares with other risks, and how homes can be modified to reduce that risk, our society should be able to cope with the problem without producing hysteria. In fact, the EPA does not suggest that a state of emergency exists when more than 4 pCi/l of radon is found in a home. Instead, it recommends that homeowners take corrective action within a few weeks or within a few years, depending on the radon level.

Professional or regulatory organizations concerned with radiation protection estimate that exposure to radon in the home in the United States results in 9,000–20,000 deaths per year. The International Committee on Radiation Protection, the first organization in the world to be officially concerned with balancing the risks of radiation against the benefits, calculates that 10,000 deaths occur each year in the United States from exposure to radon and its decay products. The National Committee on Radiation Protection, an

American organization with the same goals, estimates 9,000; the National Academy of Sciences' Committee on the Biological Effects of Ionizing Radiations, 24,000; the Nuclear Regulatory Commission (a U.S. government organization), 20,000; and the Centers for Disease Control (an organization within the U.S. government), as many as 30,000. The differences in estimates result from differences in the basic assumptions that are made, since no direct experimental data are available.

If 10,000 deaths per year result from radon-induced lung cancer, the lifetime risk to an individual from the average concentration of 1 picocurie per liter of air in the home is between 1 in 100 and 1 in 500. The risk of death from exposure to an average concentration of 8 picocuries per liter of air in the home is equal to the risk of being killed in an automobile accident in the United States. The risk of death from exposure to 100 picocuries per liter of air in the home would be equivalent to the risk of developing lung cancer from smoking a pack of cigarettes a day. Of all exposures to natural background radiation, that from radon and its decay products is the most hazardous to health. Working in a nuclear power plant exposes a worker to far less than half the radiation he or she receives from radon in the average home. People living near the Three Mile Island Nuclear plant at the time of the accident received more radiation every day from their homes than they received as a result of the accident. The maximum exposure of people living near Chernobyl at the time of the accident in the nuclear power plant was twice the exposure they will receive over their lifetime from radon. Clearly, radon and its decay products are an important source of exposure to ionizing radiation.

Should you have the radon levels measured in your house? What should you do if you are told that you have "a radon problem"? To whom can you turn for advice and help? Should you keep the problem quiet, lest the value of your property plummet? Are you likely to have to spend a lot of money to lower dangerously high radon levels?

If you decide to measure radon concentrations in your home, one of the main factors to consider is the variation in the levels from one time to another. In a single day, levels can vary by a factor of three. During different seasons, the variation may be even greater. Different parts of the house make a difference: radon concentrations in basements may be two to three times higher than those in the living areas. Whether or not windows are open during the time when the samples are obtained also is important: if the windows are open, the radon levels will be 2¹/₂ times lower than if they are kept closed. Radon levels are much higher in winter than in summer, not because the windows are closed in winter but because greater temperature gradients and drafts create a chimney effect, which decreases the pressure inside the house and draws radon from the ground into the house.

Two devices are commonly used to measure radon concentrations in a house. The first, a *track-etch detector*, filters out the alpha-emitting particles from the air over a period of a month or more, and produces microscopically visible tracks of the alpha particles on special plastic film. The second, more common device involves *charcoal absorption*. A diffusion barrier is used to keep the absorbed radon from escaping. The device, which is called a diffusion-barrier charcoal-absorption (DBCA) collector, samples the air continuously over a given period, such as a week, after which the homeowner sends the charcoal absorber to a central laboratory, where the absorbed radioactivity is measured and a report of the results is sent to the homeowner.

Contrary to popular belief, radon levels within a house do not seem to be related to the age of the house. New houses are more airtight and therefore undergo less air exchange to flush out the radon, but they are also usually built on better slab foundations, with less open earth inside the basement to allow escape of the radon from the earth. Less radon comes in, canceling out the fact that less radon goes out.

Builders sometimes wonder whether, in an effort to conserve energy by decreasing air turnover, they might make a house so airtight that a radon problem is created. Since the levels of radon in old houses are indistinguishable from those in new houses, the answer seems to be no. Insulating a house with weatherstripping or caulking, however, increases radon concentrations by about 15 percent.

Insignificant amounts of radon come from natural gas or from building materials; the major source of radon in a house is that which seeps out of the ground. Proper attention to construction methods can keep radon levels within acceptable limits.

Builders, real estate agents, and homeowners are increasingly concerned about possible radon problems that may lead to liability and litigation. They are disturbed by uncertainty, by worries about the accuracy of radon measurements, and by the lack of expertise of many of the people making the measurements. Short-term sampling can be misleading, since measurements even over a period of weeks may not accurately reflect the results that can be obtained over longer periods. Sometimes corrective measures designed to reduce radon concentrations can create problems, such as dampness or even flooding following the creation of negative pressure areas.

Builders or buyers often can't be certain whether or not there will be a radon problem after a new house is built. The situation is comparable to building a house without knowing in advance whether the septic system is going to work. It is difficult if not impossible to predict what the radon levels are likely to be in a new house from an examination of the building site before the house has been built. Insurance policies can now be obtained to cover this contingency.

Fortunately, there are readily available ways to reduce radon concentrations in a house. These include isolating basement areas that are in contact with earth, diverting soil gas by depressurization, pressurizing crawl spaces, reducing negative pressure in living areas, capping sumps, controlling cracking, and sealing cracks when they occur. Other steps include reinforcing the slab, minimizing joints in the floor, using water traps on floor drains, dampproofing exterior walls, reinforcing masonry walls to decrease cracking, running drains to daylight, and sealing off block cores. In extreme cases, one can ventilate the space beneath the slab to the outside by means of pipes extending from the crawl space to the roof, thereby creating a stack effect to vent the radon. All types of combustion within a house, such as that created in fireplaces, ovens, and furnaces, cause a negative pressure that can draw radon into a house.

Tests to screen for radon are cheap and inexpensive, and should be performed if one's basement includes a stretch of bare earth or if health department surveys reveal that there are high levels of radon in houses in the area. In such cases, the EPA recommends that sampling be made in the basement of the house after the doors and windows have been closed for twelve hours. The measurements should be made in the winter. If the radon concentration under such conditions is less than 4 picocuries per liter, there is no problem. If the level is 200 picocuries per liter or greater, the test should be repeated after several months. If the level is between 4 and 20 picocuries per liter, the test should be repeated after a year. The EPA recommends action if the level is persistently over 4 picocuries per liter. The first step in remedial action is to seal off radon entry points and increase ventilation in sump areas or below the slab in the basement.

In general, people do not seem to be as concerned about the risk of radon as about other radiation risks, perhaps because the radon question arises in the less threatening environment of the home, where people feel safe, rather than in the threatening outside world. Another factor is that the harmful effects of radon don't produce the same feelings of alienation from authority, vulnerability to the capricious actions of others, and impotence that nuclear energy seems to produce. The problem is "natural," so there is no one to blame. The same people who were up in arms over the proposed location of a uranium-waste-disposal site in New Jersey were not concerned about radon, even though the radiation exposure from the radon would have been 100 times greater than that from the uranium waste. Exposure to radon in the home can be a significant public health problem and therefore should not be underestimated—especially since there are ways to find out whether the problem exists in a given house or building and to solve the problem.

GAMMA RAYS FOR GOURMETS

A final example of radiation exposure in which perception of risk is greater than real risk is food irradiation. On September 11, 1986, mangoes from Puerto Rico appeared on the shelves of Laurenzo's Farmers Market in North Miami Beach, Florida. Above the display was a large sign that read "Treated by Irradiation." For the first time in the United States, irradiated food was being offered for sale in a grocery store. For decades, irradiation has been used to eliminate pests such as fruit flies and to extend the shelf-life of meats, fish, fruits, vegetables, and spices for days, months, or years. Some people have even called food irradiation the most important advance in nutritional health since pasteurization, but fear of radiation has prevented the food industry from making a major effort to market irradiated food, except for use in remote areas such as outer space or military installations. Two recent events brought about a rebirth of interest in supplying irradiated food to the American consumer: (1) the U.S. Environmental Protection Agency in 1985 banned the use of ethylene dibromide, a chemical fumigant used to preserve food and found to be carcinogenic in animals; and (2) the U.S. Food and Drug Administration on April 18, 1986, approved the use of irradiation to preserve fresh fruits and vegetables, extending their prior approval to irradiate herbs, spices, potatoes, wheat, wheat flour, food-grade enzymes, and pork products.

The export of mangoes had made a significant contribution to Puerto Rico's economy, but prohibition of the use of ethylene dibromide had stopped all shipments of mangoes to the United States. On hand at Laurenzo's Farmers Market on September 11, 1986, were members of the National Coalition to Stop Food Irradiation and of the Health Energy Institute, two organizations that actively oppose food irradiation and other uses of ionizing radiation. They were protesting the sale of the irradiated mangoes, charging that "food irradiation is expensive, requires further centralization of food distribution, endangers workers and the environment, and may create long-term hazards to health." The National Coalition to Stop Food Irradiation quoted from an article by J. Tevere MacFadyen in *Harrowsmith* magazine (January/February 1986): "Simply put, the proposal to establish an irradiation industry through the industrial world and the developing nations poses the greatest single technological threat to the health and welfare of the planet next to actual nuclear war."

Critics fear that radiation destroys nutrients, such as certain fats, amino acids, and vitamins A, B, C, and E, despite a lack of scientific evidence to support the claim. Other accepted food-processing techniques, particularly canning and simple overcooking, cause far greater losses of nutrients. A double standard exists in the regulatory requirements for food irradiation compared to other methods of processing food. It is well established that frying creates mutagens, for example, and grilling produces benzopyrene, a known carcinogen, yet no one has introduced legislation to ban frying or charcoal broiling.

Opponents fear that irradiated foods are potentially mutagenic and/or carcinogenic. Peroxides, considered potential carcinogens, are formed during the process of irradiation. The FDA studied the peroxide issue extensively in 1981 before permitting the use of hydrogen peroxide as a food additive for sterilizing polyethylene food packages, and concluded that there was no evidence that peroxides cause cancer. Furthermore, the level of peroxides twenty-four hours after irradiation is only about 1 part per billion, because hydrogen peroxide formed during irradiation is rapidly degraded to negligible amounts by natural enzymes and antioxidants normally present in food.

One organization, Project Cure, sponsored a direct-mail campaign to mobilize support to stop food irradiation. Project Cure generated support for a bill introduced by Congressman Douglas Bosco of California that would make food irradiation illegal. Project Cure quoted Congressman Bosco as saying: "Our government has been trying for years to figure out what to do with our radioactive nuclear waste. The . . . solution seems to be to force the American people to eat it!"

Everyone involved in the issue of food irradiation, even its opponents, acknowledges that the irradiation process does not make food radioactive, just as dental X-rays don't make your teeth radioactive. No consumer of irradiated food would be exposed to radiation. What the opponents of food irradiation say they are afraid of are unstable chemical products, called free radicals, that react with the food to create new molecules called radiolytic products. The amount of energy absorbed by the food during irradiation determines how many free radicals will be produced. According to the FDA, 100,000 rads (100 kilorad) of radiation would generate 30 parts per million of radiolytic products—that is, 0.003 percent of the food. Approximately 90 percent of these radiolytic products are known to be natural components of food; the other 10 percent have not been found in food, possibly because they are present in undetectably small amounts. These so-called unique radiolytic products are chemically similar to other natural compounds found in food.

Despite these facts, most opponents of food irradiation focus on the unique radiolytic products. According to John Gofman, one of the most prominent adversaries of all forms of nuclear technology, "The kind of epidemiological study required to find out whether or not a diet of irradiated food will increase (or possibly decrease) the frequency of cancer or genetic injuries among humans simply has not been done. . . . What is more, such a study is unlikely to ever be done, because it would require controlling the diets of 200,000 humans of various age groups for at least 50 years (preferably their full life span)."

Why is it so difficult to determine whether food irradiation is safe? The difficulty of proving that something is safe is directly related to how slight the harmful effects are. The FDA recently evaluated 413 studies on the toxicity of irradiated foods, and found that 344 were inadequate or inconclusive. Of the 69 studies it deemed to be sound scientifically, 32 suggested that there might be toxic effects, while 37 suggested that eating irradiated food was safe.

People opposed to food irradiation cite other problems that are generic to all uses of nuclear technology, such as the risks of transporting radioactive materials, possible radiation accidents in food-processing plants, and the ultimate disposal of radioactive wastes, despite the fact that the numbers of injuries, deaths, and long-term effects from accidents involving nuclear energy—both in transportation and at the worksite—are far lower than those from other industries. Irradiation facilities that use cesium-137 or cobalt-60 have been in existence for many years. In fact, they were used to irradiate disposable hospital supplies, cotton balls, feminine hygiene pads, rawhide chewbones for dogs, and baby-bottle nipples to make them sterile long before the FDA permitted the irradiation of food.

Why would anyone want to irradiate food? The World Health Organization has stated that possibly by the year 2010, nearly one billion people in the world will have access to less food than the minimum required for good health. Between 25 and 40 percent of the world's harvest is spoiled by microbes, with the greatest losses occurring in the developing countries; in tropical climates, food losses are estimated to be as high as 70 percent. The diets of many people in the developing countries of the world are deficient in both proteins and calories; the poorest people in these countries live in a chronic state of near famine. Uneven distribution of available food masks the extent and severity of these dietary inadequacies; most hunger problems are not apparent in the areas of cities visited by tourists.

Harnessing enough energy to produce sufficient food to meet

worldwide demand is one of the most important challenges facing the human race. In addition to increasing food production, we must develop technologies to improve food storage and conservation. In India, the loss of cereal grains, the major food staple, during storage accounts for about one-tenth of the country's total grain production. Before India became self-sufficient in providing grain to its population, as a result of both increased production and decreased consumption, the government spent close to $2,700 million to import 18 million tons of grain. Food irradiation has played a significant role in India's growing self-sufficiency in food production, particularly in light of the high energy costs of other methods of food preservation. Compared to all other techniques—for example, heating—irradiation consumes the smallest amount of energy. In the past, the perishable nature of fish prohibited its transport from the coasts to inland markets, and was the major obstacle to expanding the supply of seafood to the Indian population. Extending the shelf-life of fish and fruit by only a few days could prevent spoilage long enough for these products to reach their markets. Irradiation has provided the critical extension of that shelf-life, increasing demand for seafood, which in turn has stimulated the fishing industry in India.

Irradiation is used to sterilize spices that are added to processed foods and to prevent the growth of bacteria in foods to which they have been added. Irradiating spices to eliminate bacteria was approved in the United States by the FDA in 1983. About 1 percent of the spices that are used in the United States as ingredients for most processed foods have been irradiated.

The International Atomic Energy Agency (IAEA) and the Food and Agricultural Organization (FAO), both agencies of the United Nations, have held international symposia on food irradiation, drawing scientists and representatives of the food industry from all over the world. The joint IAEA-FAO-WHO Expert Committee on Wholesomeness of Irradiated Food concluded in November 1980 that irradiation of any food commodity up to an overall average dose of 1,000 kilorads presents no toxicological hazard and does not pose specific microbiological or nutritional problems.

In 1985, almost three hundred people from thirty-eight countries attended the International Symposium on Food Irradiation Processing in Washington, D.C. One year later, a similar meeting was held in Shanghai, China. Scientists presented their latest research on the irradiation of all kinds of foods from many countries, including wheat in Iraq, dried Rahu fish in Pakistan, spices in India, shrimp in the Netherlands, anchovies in Turkey, potatoes in Poland, clams in Massachusetts, and papayas in Hawaii. The attendees of the Shanghai conference concluded that within the next few years many more countries will allow food irradiation, and that ultimately international trade in irradiated food will become just as acceptable as trade in irradiated medical supplies. Eight countries (Australia, Bangladesh, Indonesia, the Republic of Korea, Malaysia, Pakistan, the Philippines, and Thailand) have established a cooperative project aimed at opening avenues of marketing and trade of irradiated foods in their region.

Irradiation facilities for treating food on a commercial scale are in operation in twenty-eight countries, including Belgium, Hungary, Australia, Bulgaria, Chile, Czechoslovakia, Denmark, France, Israel, Italy, the Netherlands, the Philippines, South Africa, the Soviet Union, Spain, Thailand, the United Kingdom, Uruguay, and West Germany. In September 1987, twenty-seven new irradiation facilities were under construction (or in an advanced planning stage) for the commercial treatment of food. Japan irradiates 10,000 tons of potatoes per year to inhibit sprouting. The Netherlands has been especially active in using food irradiation; at a plant in the city of Ede, about 70–85 tons of food are irradiated every week, mainly spices, marine products, egg powders, and dried vegetables treated to control microbes. (Fresh agricultural products are not irradiated in the Netherlands.) In the Soviet Union, hundreds of thousands of tons of grain have been disinfected by irradiation at the plant in Odessa.

Why has food irradiation caught on so slowly in the United States, especially since American scientists in the 1940s pioneered the technology? The U.S. government approved a limited use of irradiation for potatoes and wheat flour in the 1960s, but the food industry has shied away from investing in irradiation plants. The main reason is that the government and the food industry believe that the general public would be afraid to buy irradiated food because of their perception of the risk of radiation. Ironically, it was the risk of cancer from chemical food additives, such as ethylene dibromide and sodium nitrite, that steered the food industry toward irradiation as an alternative means of food preservation. The rising costs of the energy needed for other forms of food preservation and storage have also made food irradiation more attractive. It is estimated that food irradiation costs only half as much as fumigating with ethylene dibromide.

In some cases, food irradiation may be more costly than other preservation techniques. A company may have food-packaging plants spread out all over the country, and may not want to incur the costs of shipping food to a centralized irradiation facility. Nevertheless, it is likely that the food industry would at times choose food irradiation if it believed that the public would accept it.

One of the most hotly contested issues in the irradiation debate is the labeling of irradiated foods. Originally, the FDA proposed that foods not be identified as irradiated, but in April 1986, the agency stipulated that foods must carry a label with the wording "treated with irradiation," accompanied by the international symbol for food irradiation. Those who oppose this type of labeling believe that it misleads consumers, making them afraid of a danger that does not exist. Other terms, such as "ionized fresh" and "picowaved," have been proposed, but they sound like attempts to meet labeling requirements without letting the vast majority of food shoppers know that the food has been irradiated. Some restaurateurs question whether they'll eventually have to indicate on menus whether the food they serve has been irradiated. Processed foods that contain irradiated spices do not have to carry the label. Currently, the FDA requires that irradiated products sold to wholesalers be marked "Treated with Radiation. Do Not Irradiate Again."

In February 1985, *Good Housekeeping* magazine surveyed 100 middle-class married women in Philadelphia and asked whether they would prefer that food spoilage be retarded by chemical preservatives or by irradiation. Only 3 percent said they would choose chemical preservatives, whereas 23 percent said they would prefer irradiation. Of the remaining women, 44 percent said they did not know enough to judge and 27 percent wanted neither method. In August 1986, *Good Housekeeping* published an article on food irradiation, describing how the process can kill insects, molds, or harmful bacteria that can lead to spoilage—even illness. The article stated that as a result of the FDA's recent approval of the irradiation of fresh fruits, vegetables, and mushrooms, "You'll probably be seeing more irradiated foods in your market," and food prices may actually go down because of the resulting decrease in spoilage.

In response to the article, the magazine received about twenty-five letters of complaint—including one letter accusing *Good Housekeeping* of supporting food irradiation because of an alliance with the devil. Considering that about five million women read *Good Housekeeping*, the small number of complaints may indicate that American homemakers are ready to accept food irradiation. Eventually, if consumers accept "ionized fresh" foods, they may also decide that the labeling requirement is an unnecessary cost.

Irradiated food may be something new to most Americans, but for many years it has been served to cancer patients recovering from bone-marrow transplants. According to the director of clinical nutrition at one hospital, "Irradiation leaves the food more palatable than alternatives such as autoclaving, thus helping the patients regain their appetites, a prerequisite to discharge from the hospital." The Apollo astronauts of the 1960s also ate irradiated food during space flights. It is possible that someday everyone on earth will eat it from time to time without a second thought.

David Laurenzo, vice-president of Laurenzo's Farmers Market in North Miami Beach, where the first irradiated food was commercially sold in the United States, reported that the twenty cases of mangoes (at $1.49 per pound) were quickly snapped up by shoppers. "The people who are buying the mangoes are mango lovers. It [doesn't] seem to matter to them if they are irradiated or not."

5

THE SEARCH
FOR TRUTH

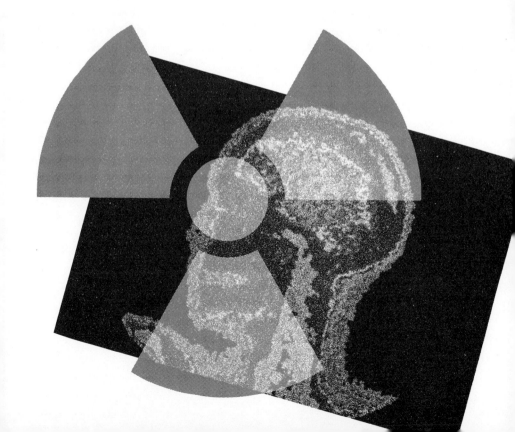

Above all, if any man could succeed—not in merely bringing to light one particular invention, however useful—but in kindling in nature a luminary which would, at its first rising, shed some light on the present limits and borders of human discoveries . . . it seemed to me that such a discoverer would deserve to be called the true extender of the Kingdom of Man over the universe, the Champion of human liberty.

Francis Bacon (1561–1616)

Preceding page: A brain scan following the injection of a radioactive tracer. Prepared in collaboration with Jonathon Links.

FIGHTING IGNORANCE AND FEAR

Life is a process of continuous change. To live is to change. To change is to be uncertain. To be uncertain is to experience anxiety and fear. Reality is a process of continuous change and bewildering complexity. Resisting change may bring about contentment in the short run, but we risk losing touch with reality. Ignorance may be bliss, but it can also be dangerous.

Human beings view change as a threat because the human brain evolved at a time when wild animals might lunge out of the forest and attack at any time. Fear and aggression saved our ancestors. The instinctive choice of "fight or flight" became programed into the human genetic code, making possible adaptations that allowed our species to evolve and survive. Over hundreds of thousands of years of primitive life, human behavior was progressively modified by lessons taught to generation after generation of ancestors. Sensory, emotional, and behavioral experiences over eons shaped our genetic makeup.

In our modern, civilized society, overt aggression and cowardly retreat at a personal level have become socially unacceptable, but we accept the concept of a "just" war. Though far from perfect, the scientific method is an antidote to ignorance, fear, and agression.

Adopting the scientific method requires modesty, character, and honesty. We must be modest enough to accept the fact that we do not know everything and we must continually search for more information; we must have enough character to seek the truth even when we fear we won't like it; and we must be able to accept new views that contradict what we believed previously. Each of us must decide whether science and technology are the causes or the cures of present-day problems, and whether the scientific method remains the most effective way to deal with the increasing dangers of violence and destructive behavior.

Aristotle, the Greek philosopher of the fourth century B.C., taught us how to apply deductive reasoning to the solution of our problems. He paved the way for the invention of the scientific method as we know it today.

Galileo Galilei was born on February 14, 1564, in Pisa, Italy. His observations of the movements of the stars and planets with the newly invented telescope led him to conclude that the earth was not the center of the universe. As has often been the case throughout history, the invention of a new instrument brought advances in human knowledge. Galileo's careful observations and new ideas revolutionized not only the field of astronomy but also that of philosophy. When Galileo concluded that the earth revolves around the sun, this new view of the universe frightened established authorities. Eventually his views prevailed, and his invention of the scientific method opened the human mind to a whole new way of looking at natural phenomena. Prior to the time of Galileo, many ancient civilizations had developed advanced technologies, but the concept of scientific investigation was a giant leap forward for the human race. After the discovery of Galileo's law of free-falling bodies, other natural laws were promulgated, including Johannes Kepler's law of planetary motions, Isaac Newton's law of gravity, Robert Boyle's law of gases, René Descartes's law of refraction, and Gregor Mendel's law of heredity. In the seventeenth century, Newton, the British mathematician, scientist, and philosopher, added differential calculus and mathematical theory to the scientific method, thus going beyond experiments and observations. Mathematical logic (deductive reasoning based on observations) made it possible to see otherwise obscure relationships between observed results. Albert Einstein's theory of relativity is an example of mathematical derivations based on the observations of other scientists.

The scientific method can be used by just about anyone, and provides an effective way to approach the problems of everyday life. Children can be taught to be skeptical yet open minded, can be encouraged to say "Show me" or "Prove it." A curious child who pushes the lid off a dusty box in a corner of the attic is learning how to conduct an experiment. Observing what's inside the box is better than simply guessing. As infants and children, we learn to observe and draw conclusions. After our childhood years, we tend to become more and more rigid, dogmatic, and narrow-minded in our thinking. We lose the curiosity we possessed as children, the open-mindedness that characterizes the lifelong student. We adopt rigid habits of thought that serve as a defense against the anxiety of change and uncertainty, but that at times can cause problems.

In adopting a scientific approach to problem solving, we try to: (1) ask clear questions; (2) search for patterns and relationships in our observations, whenever possible describing the relationships in quantitative terms; (3) design experiments to test our ability to make correct predictions; (4) observe natural phenomena under experimentally altered conditions; (5) confirm or modify our beliefs on the basis of the new observations; and (6) repeat the process to determine whether the results are reproducible.

HOW TO CHOOSE: RISK PERCEPTION AND RISK ASSESSMENT

Given the increasing complexity of modern life, it is no wonder that we often feel confused. Scientific news tends to be highly specialized. We are presented with new discoveries and changing views so rapidly that we begin to believe that nothing remains "true" for very long. We may develop a cynical attitude. If currently held scientific tenets will eventually be disproved, why believe anything?

Continual scientific controversies bewilder the public. Stories of scientific fraud damage the credibility of the scientific community and the scientific method in the public's eyes. Nevertheless, the best antidote to fear is knowledge, which can help us distinguish legitimate from exaggerated fears. Science continues to provide an increasingly realistic view of the world, and can help us decide which risks to take and which to ignore.

In their book *Risk and Culture*, Mary Douglas and Aaron Wildavsky stated: "Choice depends upon alternatives, values, and beliefs. . . . Values and uncertainties are an integral part of every acceptable-risk problem. . . . There are no value-free processes for choosing between risky alternatives. The search for an 'objective method' [of assessing the acceptability of risk] is doomed to failure and may blind the searchers to the value-laden assumptions they are making." The issue is, "who should rule and what should matter."

An example of erroneous perception of risk occurred at the time of the accident at the Chernobyl nuclear power plant. An estimated 100,000–200,000 pregnant women throughout Western Europe were so frightened by the possible adverse effects of radiation on their unborn children that they had abortions even though they wanted to give birth to their babies—and even though the levels of radiation exposure from Chernobyl in Western Europe were nowhere near the levels associated with birth defects. Andrea Bianco, of the International Atomic Energy Agency in Vienna, said that "pregnancies have been interrupted with the wrong advice of medical doctors, who knew very little, or only in a distorted way, about radiation." Hundreds of thousands of women mistakenly believed they were sparing themselves and their families the heartache of caring for a child with birth defects.

What facts were available to help these women make this critically important decision? What do we know about the risks of radiation? First, everyone should be aware that scientists all over the world have been carrying out extensive studies of the biological effects of ionizing radiation for more than fifty years. The International Commission on Radiological Protection (ICRP) was established in 1928 in response to the growing use of X-rays and radium in medical practice. Its goal was to inform radiologists about radiation protection and to promote the safe and effective use of these new medical procedures. The commission has an official relationship with the World Health Organization (WHO) and the International Atomic Energy Agency (IAEA). It also maintains a close working relationship with the U.N. Scientific Committee on the Effects of Atomic Radiation (UNSCEAR). This committee provides the ICRP with scientific data from research performed throughout the world, collaborates in making recommendations on maximum permissible levels of radiation exposure for workers and the general public, and promotes safe radiological practices. The ICRP is composed of a chairman and not more than twelve other members who are chosen on the basis of their internationally recognized expertise, their experience and research contributions in the fields of medical radiology, public health, epidemiology, radiation physics and protection, physics, health physics, biophysics, genetics, and radiation dosimetry. Nominations for membership are made by scientific societies throughout the world. The ICRP continually evaluates radiation research and publishes reports. In 1955, the United

Nations formed the UNSCEAR, which reviews worldwide scientific data on human exposure to ionizing radiation. In addition, countless research institutions and federal agencies conduct studies of the effects of radiation, which are reviewed by other scientists and published in the scientific literature.

The first standards for permissible levels of radiation exposure for workers and the general public were recommended in 1928 and were subsequently reevaluated in 1931, 1934, 1937, 1951, 1955, 1959, 1977, 1980, and 1985. Most estimates of risk from exposure to low doses of radiation (below 50 rads) are extrapolated from the observed increased incidence of disease resulting from higher doses of radiation exposure. The maximum permissible level of exposure for the general public—500 millirems per year—was adopted in 1958, and remained unchanged until 1977, when it was reduced to 100 millirems per year. At its meeting in March 1985, the ICRP reaffirmed this level, while stating that a level of 500 millirems per year was permissible provided the average annual effective dose over the individual's lifetime did not exceed 100 millirems.

Initially, the limitations to radiation exposure were based on concern over its possible genetic effects. Today, the role of radiation in increasing the incidence of cancer is the major concern. In addressing these concerns, it is important to remember that life on earth evolved in the presence of background ionizing radiation. Manufactured radiation has the potential of increasing the number of mutations occurring naturally, but to date, no data obtained from human beings have revealed a measurable increase in the number of mutations resulting from radiation. Low doses of radiation do not increase the number of detectable mutations that occur in human beings. Genetic effects have been produced in experimental organisms and in plants, but it is not known whether these results can be extrapolated to human beings. From studies involving millions of mice, researchers have calculated that the amount of radiation that would be needed to double the natural or spontaneous mutation rate is between 20 and 200 rems. Agencies concerned with radiation protection, such as the ICRP and the National Research Council of the United States, accept the principle that most mutations are harmful, and contend that any dose of radiation, however small, entails some genetic risk.

The survivors of the atomic bombings at Hiroshima and Nagasaki constitute the largest group of human beings that has been studied for the effects of exposure to manufactured radiation. Detailed studies of two generations of descendants of these survivors have revealed no increase in the incidence of prenatal or neonatal deaths, or in the frequency of malformations, despite the fact that the average dose of radiation to which their parents and grandparents were exposed was 100 rems.

On the other hand, there is no doubt that radiation can cause cancer. The question is, what is the degree of risk? How much does radiation exposure increase the risk of cancer? Unfortunately, it is not possible to obtain accurate estimates of risk to human beings from studies of animals exposed to radiation. In many cases, the animals are highly inbred and genetically predisposed to develop leukemia or other forms of cancer.

Data have been obtained from human populations, however, such as the atomic bomb survivors and persons exposed to medical or occupational radiation. Included in the latter group are radiologists, radium-dial painters, uranium miners, shipyard workers, persons injected with radioactive thorium (Thorotrast) in diagnostic X-ray procedures, and patients treated for scalp infections, ankylosing spondylitis (a form of arthritis), or enlargement of the thymus gland.

From the study of these populations, numerous attempts have been made to assess the risk resulting from exposure to low doses of radiation. An important question is whether there is a certain dose of radiation below which no harm will occur to the exposed human being—that is, below which there is no additional risk of that person's developing cancer. The existence of such a "threshold" cannot be proved or disproved. It can be claimed only on the basis of an educated guess, on what happens to people who are exposed to higher doses of radiation. Beyond question, in large groups of people who are exposed to doses of 50–100 rems, an excess number of cancers will occur above the number expected normally. The problem arises in interpreting whether the risk at high doses can be extrapolated, or extended, down to low doses, such as 10 rems or less.

The assumption that the relationship between dose and effect (in producing cancer) is linear for low doses as well as high doses is known as the "linear hypothesis." The dictionary tells us that a hypothesis is "an unproved theory, proposition, supposition, etc., tentatively accepted to explain certain facts or to provide a basis for further investigation, argument, etc." On the basis of a hypothesis, scientists design further experiments to try to find out whether the assumption is correct. If further experiments do not support the hypothesis, then it is abandoned. The linear hypothesis is supported by studies of patients with thyroid and breast cancer down to levels of exposure to radiation in the range of 6–16 rems. Acceptance of the "linear–no threshold hypothesis" would lead to the prediction that whole-body exposure of 10,000 persons to 1 rem of X-rays, gamma rays, or beta particles would result in one additional cancer death in that population. But that one person's death could never be detected, because it would have to be included in the deaths of the 2,700 persons of the group who would die from cancer from *all* causes, mostly unknown causes.

These values are calculated by assuming that the number of cases will be exactly proportional to the radiation dosage at all levels. Some scientists reject this premise, believing that there are no adverse health effects from exposures of less than 10 rads. It is impossible to determine the existence or nonexistence of a "threshold dose" below which there is no increased risk, however; if the excess risk is truly proportional to the dose, and if 1,000 exposed and 1,000 control subjects are required to test the risk adequately at 100 rems, then about 100,000 people in each group would be required to test the risk of 10 rems, and about 10 million people in each group would be required to determine the risk of 1 rem per person.

Most of the estimates of the risk from exposure to low-level ionizing radiation have been based on the examination of the 113,169 survivors of the atomic bombings of Hiroshima and Nagasaki. For decades after the bombings, researchers assumed that almost all the exposure at Nagasaki had been due to gamma radiation (the type received in medical and occupational exposures), while that at Hiroshima included about 23–35 percent neutron irradiation. There is now evidence that this assumption was incorrect, and that the neutron dose at Hiroshima was much lower, because of the shielding effects of buildings and humid weather conditions. Between 1950 and 1969, 88 new cases of leukemia were observed in Hiroshima; only 29 were reported in Nagasaki. Because of the supposed neutron dosage at Hiroshima, the Nagasaki data were used to estimate the risk of medical and occupational radiation exposure. The newest calculations include the Hiroshima leukemia cases as well, since researchers now believe that the exposure there also was due primarily to gamma radiation.

Other controversial studies include that by T. Mancuso, A. Stewart, and G. Kneale (1977), who found a higher-than-expected incidence of cancer in radiation workers at the Hanford plutonium-reprocessing plant in Richland, Washington, where radiation exposure was close to one rem. These investigators estimated that exposure to one rem increased the risk of all forms of cancer by 8 percent (125 percent for bone marrow cancers), but their data did not show a dose-related increase in the incidence of leukemia. Several other studies have criticized these findings, claiming inadequate measurement of radiation exposure and the presence of other carcinogens. The conclusions of the Mancuso study were not accepted by the National Academy of Sciences' Committee on the Biological Effects of Ionizing Radiations (BEIR committee) in its 1980 report.

T. Najarian and T. Colton (1978) concluded from responses to interviews that the incidence of cancer, including leukemia, was increased in shipyard workers in Portsmouth, New Hampshire. The BEIR committee rejected this study as well, noting that it "provides a remarkable illustration of the dangers of response bias in epidemiological studies."

Scientists and others concerned with establishing guidelines for safe levels of radiation exposure chose the linear hypothesis so that if they were wrong, the risk from radiation would be overestimated rather than underestimated. This is often referred to as a "conservative approach," in that its advocates expect the worst situation to be the true situation. It is important to remember, however, that the real risk from low doses of radiation may be much lower than that predicted by the linear hypothesis, or even nonexistent. When decisions must be made concerning low-level radiation, it is important to distinguish fact from hypothesis. For example, legal issues should be based on evidence, not hypotheses. On the other hand, radiation exposure, even at low doses, should be kept as low as reasonably achievable in designing radiation workplaces or storage facilities.

Many people totally reject any human activities that result in an increase in environmental radiation above background, or naturally occurring, levels. They tend to overlook the fact that compared to other risks of daily life, such as those incurred from poverty, malnutrition, infections, handguns, automobile crashes, household and industrial accidents, smoking cigarettes, drug abuse, urban crime, and natural catastrophes, the risks from low levels of ionizing radiation are small indeed. Deep-sea fishing, coal mining, working in an oil refinery, and construction work are all risky—far more risky than working with medical radiation or in a nuclear power plant. Smoking cigarettes, being 30 percent overweight, or consuming excessive amounts of alcohol is riskier than exposure to low levels of radiation. Tornadoes, hurricanes, floods, and earthquakes kill far more people than ionizing radiation does.

Moreover, fear of low-level radiation is linked to fear of cancer-causing agents in general—toxic chemicals, for instance. Many people believe that most cancers are caused either by radiation or by manufactured chemical substances in the environment. They believe that the 27 percent of us who die from cancer need not do so. Such beliefs are encouraged by publications like that of the National Institute for Occupational Safety and Health, *Suspected Carcinogens* (1976), which lists 2,413 carcinogenic substances. Newspaper headlines continually warn us of the threat of cancer associated with charcoal-broiled meats, coffee, beer, food additives, magnetic fields from electric power lines, chemicals, and radiation. Common household paper products, including disposable diapers, have been found to contain traces of dioxin, a substance that can produce cancer in laboratory animals. Joe Jackson, a popular singer, recently recorded a song called "Everything Causes Cancer."

Science and technology are no longer automatically accepted as beneficial to society. They have become more and more a source of fear and concern. Mistrust of technology has been institutionalized in hundreds of organizations that, with a sense of dedication to what they believe is the public interest, promulgate the idea that chemical and radioactive carcinogens are widespread and at times imply that their use reflects immoral behavior motivated by economic and political greed. Such mistrust has engendered exaggerated fear of exposure to carcinogens (substances causing cancer), mutagens (substances causing genetic abnormalities), and teratogens (substances causing fetal abnormalities).

Some scientists, including Philip Handler, former president of the National Academy of Sciences, point out that we in industrialized societies are suffering not from an epidemic of cancer but from an epidemic of life. The increased rates of cancer reflect the fact that more people are living to the advanced ages at which cancer has always been prevalent. In industrialized countries, the overall age-corrected incidence of cancer has not in fact increased, but has actually been declining slowly. According to Handler, only a tiny fraction of all current deaths due to cancer—in the United States or elsewhere—are due to manufactured chemicals. Only 1-2 percent of all cases of cancer can be traced to occupational exposure in such workplaces as coal mines, asbestos mines, and factories. Pollutants in general are said to contribute to no more than about 5 percent of all cancers. The causes of most types of cancer remain unknown.

Risks become intolerable when people begin to think they can escape them. Because so many former problems of pregnancy and childbirth have been overcome, for example, most people expect every baby to be born healthy. Many parents look for a culprit when their baby is born sick or deformed, not realizing that genetic disorders of unknown cause still affect about 10 percent of all live-born babies. Disorders—including congenital malformations, mental retardation, dwarfism, and diseases such as sickle cell anemia, diabetes, cystic fibrosis, hemophilia, and muscular dystrophy—remain important causes of human misery and warrant ongoing commitments to further scientific research. We should be concerned about hazardous substances, and attempt to decrease their health risks, but we must continue to channel the lion's share of available research time and money into efforts to solve major health problems. The amount of time, energy, and money a society spends to solve its problems should be proportional to the amount of damage caused by those problems.

For example, cigarette smoking causes more premature deaths in the United States than do any of the following: AIDS, cocaine, heroin, alcohol, fires, automobile accidents, homicides, and suicides. Yet questionable carcinogens make the headlines, and find their way into legislation and lawsuits. The attainment of a tobacco-free society by the year 2000 would produce a gain in life expectancy comparable to the complete elimination of all cancers not caused by tobacco use. Nevertheless, many people go on worrying and smoking.

One way to allocate resources to each problem is to consider the cost per life saved. Dr. Bernard L. Cohen, a radiation expert at the University of Pittsburgh, has estimated that removing radon from drinking water to levels recommended as safe by the U.S. Environmental Protection Agency (EPA) would cost $5 million per life saved. Cancer screening would cost about $100,000 per life saved. Reducing radon levels in houses to meet EPA guidelines would cost about $23,000 per life saved. According to Dr. Cohen, "With this perspective, it is difficult to see how one can question the cost-effectiveness of the $23,000 per life saved being spent on the problem of indoor radon in homes."

If a major city in the northeastern United States became as obsessed with the dangers from tornadoes as it was with radiation and changed its building codes and developed evacuation plans, allocating funds to this project that were disproportionate to the monies it spent for handgun control, crime prevention, drug abuse, highway safety, and education, most people would agree that the community was not using its resources wisely. By this we do not imply that the risks of radiation should be ignored. Rather, we would argue that the risks should be addressed more realistically. The public is often confused, not because people lack intelligence, but because they do not have an adequate understanding of what is known about radiation, what is unknown, and what is speculation. A very astute person once said, "It ain't what we don't know that hurts us; it's what we know that ain't so."

People are willing to incur far greater risks during voluntary activities (witness cigarette smoking or hang gliding or even sunbathing) than when they believe (1) that they have no choice and (2) that the risk is imposed on them by others. For example, sunbathing for long periods is a widespread practice, despite its well-known side effects: burning, aging of the skin, increased risk of skin cancer, damage to the eyes, alterations of the immune system, and even allergies. Basal- and squamous-cell carcinoma of the skin are clearly caused by exposure to the ultraviolet portions of the electromagnetic radiation from the sun, ultraviolet B being the most harmful. The mechanism of injury of ultraviolet radiation is damage to nucleic acids and proteins in DNA, which can cause cross-linking or single strand breaks in the DNA molecules. It is probable that malignant melanoma also is caused by exposure of the skin to sunlight. Despite the recommendations by physicians and organizations, including the American Medical Association, that we minimize our exposure to the sun and use sunscreens, most people ignore the warnings, accept the risks, and sunbathe anyway.

The use of tanning machines was particularly dangerous in the past, because the early models emitted essentially the harmful form of radiation, ultraviolet B. In recent years, however, newer types of tanning booths and beds have been designed to emit primarily ultraviolet A radiation. This development has increased the public's interest in such apparatuses, particularly in areas where natural sunlight is less prevalent—for instance, in Scandinavia. The U.S. Food and Drug Administration has imposed specific requirements for the design and use of tanning devices, but it is possible to operate the machines without conforming to the guidelines. Other than their cosmetic and psychological effects, the only benefit of such machines is their conversion of 7-dehydrocholesterol to vitamin D3.

Woven into the involuntary aspect of radiation exposure are political issues. The inhabitants of the Marshall Islands were exposed to radiation by a foreign country that occupied their territory after World War II. The Navaho Indians of the southwestern United States were exposed to radiation from uranium mines and uranium mill tailings coming from the industry that was built by the Caucasian peoples who conquered the North American Indian nations. Some villagers in Bukit Merah believe that valuable rare earths are being taken from them and shipped to Japan, while the toxic residues from the mining of these elements are being left behind to contaminate their land and water.

No one can deny that at times the perceived risk is less than the real risk. When this is the case, people may not do what is necessary to reduce the risk. On the other hand, when the perceived risk is far greater than the real risk, people spend a lot of time, energy, and money trying to reduce the imagined risk, neglecting or minimizing the real risk in the process. There is a growing tendency to refuse to accept risks that have been considered acceptable in the past. More and more people seek to blame a person, a company, or the government for putting them at risk.

Today radiation is a major source of fear worldwide for a lot a reasons. It is invisible and cannot be detected by our sense of smell, taste, hearing, or touch. Radiation burst into our collective consciousness as the atomic bomb. To most people, radiation is a poorly understood human-made force for evil.

Education is one way to battle that fear. In the words of Thomas Jefferson, "I know no safe depository of the ultimate powers of society but the people themselves; and if we think them not enlightened enough to exercise their control with a wholesome discretion, the remedy is not to take it from them but to inform their discretion." Education of the public must be a goal of the people concerned with extracting the benefits of radiation for humankind while minimizing the risks.

EPILOGUE

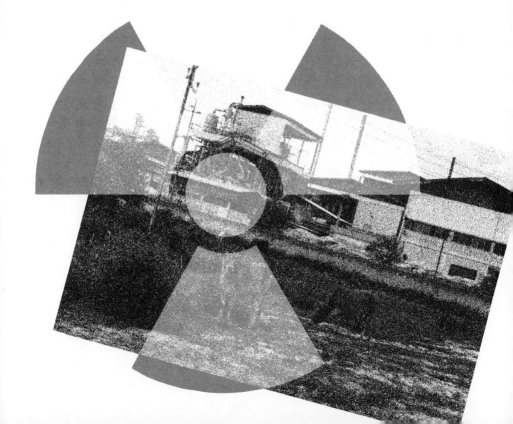

Have you ever thought that war is a madhouse and that everyone in a war is a patient?

Oriana Fallaci, 1972

From the moment of conception until long after we are dead, each of us is constantly exposed to radiation from many sources: from cosmic rays that filter through the atmosphere; from uranium-238 and its decay products in the soil; and from radioactivity within our bodies. One of every ten thousand potassium atoms in the human body is radioactive. The earth's atmosphere shields us from some cosmic radiation. People who live at higher altitudes have less atmospheric protection and therefore more exposure to radiation than people who live at sea level. Residents of Colorado are exposed to about twice as much natural background radiation as people living in Florida. Airplane pilots and flight attendants are exposed to higher than normal levels of radiation because of the time they spend at higher altitudes. Some receive such high doses that technically they should be designated as "radiation workers."

If we cannot escape ionizing radiation, where should we draw the line? Should we try to limit our exposure to "natural" radiation? Should we avoid all types of manufactured ionizing radiation? Are present standards of acceptable levels of radiation exposure adequate? Is nuclear technology inherently too dangerous to be used for anything? Do the nonmilitary uses of radiation increase or decrease the risk of a nuclear holocaust? Is any exposure to manufactured radiation worth the risk?

There are no easy answers to these questions, but we have to confront them, and we should begin to teach our children and grandchildren about microcuries, becquerels, rads, and rems just as we teach them about meters, kilograms, and seconds. We have to teach them about the biological effects and risks of manufactured radiation, and then let them decide whether the benefits of specific activities are greater than the risks.

Reality and the perception of reality are often far apart. We would all be a lot better off if we brought the two closer together. Some members of our species have chosen to produce enough nuclear weapons to destroy the earth, believing, presumably, that the benefits exceed the risks. Others believe that the risks of nuclear war now far exceed the risks inherent in abolishing all nuclear weapons. Still others want to decrease the number of nuclear weapons, but not completely eliminate them.

For most people, an annihilating nuclear war, whether planned or accidental, is too depressing to contemplate. No one can really imagine what a nuclear holocaust would be like, and so some have chosen to devote all their energies to the elimination of all uses of radiation, believing that by doing this they reduce the risk of nuclear war.

Undoubtedly, fear can be helpful. For example, after a heart attack, a person is often able to stop smoking, lose weight, and change his or her lifestyle dramatically, while this behavior was not possible before the heart attack. However, the fear of nuclear war can at times cloud a person's thinking and decisions about the benefits of radiation.

We know that we are neither smarter nor morally better than our forebears, who at the close of World War II were the first human beings to try to balance the benefits against the risks of developing atomic energy. We have the advantage of hindsight, however, for we have witnessed the nuclear arms race that was so feared by that generation.

Unwarranted fear can be a major problem and, indeed, may be the major factor in the continuation of the nuclear arms race. Just as fear of the insane led to chains, iron cages, and strait jackets in the asylums of the nineteenth century, fear has put the human race in the strait jacket of nuclear weapons. Just as strait jackets made the mentally ill more violent, so too the existence of nuclear weapons has increased the probability that they will be used violently. Is there not danger in the policy that the United States will continue to build nuclear weapons, in the words of President Reagan, to "the point that no other nation on this earth will ever dare to raise a hand against us, and in this way we will preserve world peace?" Such an approach risks a violent response. Violence in insane asylums was eliminated by the unvarying kindness of Phillippe Pinel and other early psychiatrists. Nonrestraint became the principle in caring for the mentally ill. Can the same philosophy decrease the likelihood of nuclear war?

One of the greatest paradoxes of all time is that nuclear radiation is likely to be our salvation. Radioactive tracers may be what it takes to increase our understanding of the emotions of fear, violence, and destructiveness to the point that we can diminish the dangers of nuclear war. PET (positron emission tomography) studies of the human brain can help us understand better the chemistry of fear, aggression, and violence, so that we can direct our energies in safe and constructive directions toward further human progress rather than a nuclear holocaust. The solution to the dangers of the atomic nucleus may lie in the exploration of the chemistry of human emotions, the chemistry of fear, paranoia, and aggression.

Many people underestimate the risks and dangers of nuclear war, and overestimate the risks of the peaceful uses of atomic energy. They seek to block the development of all applications of nuclear radiation, including the peaceful uses of atomic energy. They do not accept the premise that radiation can be adequately controlled and used safely for the benefit of the human species. They do not distinguish sufficiently between the benefits of its peaceful uses and the destructive effects of its military uses.

Aggressive behavior seems to be built into human genes, and is encouraged daily by environmental forces. Linked to that aggression is fear. Both emotions are thought to be reflected in measurable changes in the chemistry of the brain. If we find chemical changes related to fear and violence, we may be better able to control their occurrence. We need a better understanding of the workings of the human mind, and radioactive tracers can now help us achieve that in ways that physicists, chemists, and political leaders at the end of World War II only dreamed of.

In the developing countries of the world, poverty, malnutrition, and infectious diseases—particularly cholera and malaria—remain the major sources of misery and death. In Malaysia, for instance, vehicular accidents, tuberculosis, malaria, and hepatitis are the major causes of sickness and death, and their risk is far greater than the risk of radiation-induced cancer or genetic defects associated with the operation of the Asian Rare Earth plant in Bukit Merah. The underdeveloped countries' most pressing problems can be solved only by economic development and better distribution of the world's resources. If the highly developed countries continue to use the major part of the world's oil supply to provide energy, how will the developing countries raise their standards of living? How much longer will the developing countries continue to accept the status quo?

Medical X-ray procedures help practically everyone in industrialized societies at one time or another, and at times they even save people's lives, but the fear of low-level radiation may inhibit the use of medical radiation in the future. If a poll were taken today, many people would describe themselves as "antinuclear." The question is, are they against nuclear war, nuclear weapons, nuclear power, nuclear medicine, nuclear agriculture, the nuclear industry? Are they antinuclear everything? The philosophy of some is that though we can produce radioactivity, we cannot destroy it; and since it is harmful, we should not produce any more.

All of us are concerned about the future of our children and our grandchildren, but we need not accept the fatalistic view: "Forget human survival and adjust psychologically to the death of the human species as we must adjust to the death of a human being." Instead, we can choose to believe that the human race will one day be able to break with its violent past, despite countless failures, and that human ignorance, not science, is the problem. Perhaps one day we will heed the words of the American Indian Chief Joseph, who at the end of a lifetime of warfare declared, "I will fight no more forever," or the words of another great American leader, Martin Luther King, Jr., who believed that one day "the brotherhood of men will become a reality."

On December 7, 1987, President Ronald Reagan and General Secretary Mikhail Gorbachev signed the first agreement ever to eliminate an entire class of nuclear weapons: 859 American and 1,752 Soviet intermediate and short-range missiles. This reduction could be the forerunner of further cuts in the superpowers' long-range nuclear weapons. General Secretary Gorbachev called the treaty "the first step down the road leading to a nuclear-free world." Declaring that "we are living in a time of new reality," he appealed to the American people to press their political leaders to seize what he described as a "historic opportunity to improve East-West relations."

Although the missiles that are to be removed represent only 4 percent of the superpowers' total nuclear arsenal, this could indeed be a first step on the road to nuclear disarmament. Ratification of the treaty could pave the way to the next stage—an agreement to reduce long-range nuclear weapons by 50 percent, limiting both sides to 4,900 nuclear warheads on land-based and sea-launched ballistic missiles. In light of the agreement reached in December 1987, the board of directors of the *Bulletin of Atomic Scientists*, a journal founded forty years ago by a group of nuclear scientists that included Albert Einstein and J. Robert Oppenheimer, moved the hands of the "Doomsday Clock" three more minutes back from midnight, to 11:54 P.M., because the actions of the superpower leaders had lessened the threat of nuclear war. It was the first time in sixteen years that the symbolic indicator of the imminence of nuclear war had been moved back. The hands on the clock were last moved forward in December 1983, after arms control efforts at that time failed.

Advances in the direction of peace are also being made at the scientific level. At the conclusion of a conference entitled "Peace through Mind/Brain Research," held in Hamamatsu City, Japan, from April 29 to May 3, 1988, leading scientists and engineers from Japan, the Soviet Union, and the United States reached an agreement to develop a joint mind/brain program to facilitate research directed toward an understanding of the relationship between the human brain and human behavior. A research center will be built at Hamamatsu City to take advantage of major advances in positron emission tomography and other photonics technology, including laser tomography. Academician A. M. Prokhorov, leader of the Soviet delegation to the conference and recipient of the Nobel Prize in physics in 1964 for his research on lasers, stated in an opening message: "I am convinced that further development and enhancement of scientific collaboration among Soviet, Japanese and American scientists will strengthen governmental relationships. Their research will require not only the creation of a research institute, but also their concentrated and mutual efforts."

In another message to the conference, Dr. D. A. Henderson, dean of the Johns Hopkins School of Public Health and Hygiene and recipient of the 1988 Japan Prize for his work in eliminating smallpox, commented, "We fully anticipate that through closer collaborative efforts of Japanese scientists and engineers, together with American and Soviet scientists, we can substantially advance a critical new area of science and the cause of world peace."

Mr. Teruo Hiruma, president of Hamamatsu Photonics, stated that "the language of science is the same for people all over the world. The road to peace will be through mind/brain science."

Violence—both personal and cultural—may not be uncontrollable or inevitable. Perhaps one day it will be regarded as aberrant national as well as personal behavior, a disease similar to mental illnesses.

After World War II, many people assumed that a broad development of the peaceful uses of nuclear energy would help eliminate its warlike uses. Scientists and political leaders hoped that the use of atomic energy to generate electricity and to advance biomedical research would decrease the likelihood of nuclear war and help control the development of nuclear weapons. They thought that the development of peaceful uses would attract "the best human resources of good will, imagination, and ingenuity," people who would then be in a position to help solve the problem of a nuclear arms race.

A highlight of 1946 was the first shipment of a radioactive substance from the Manhattan District atomic bomb project to a hospital. This substance was a forerunner of the radioactive tracers now used for biomedical and other scientific research in universities and research laboratories all over the world. The same year marked the invention of the Univac digital computer, which was able to carry out 5,000 calculations per second—nothing compared to the capabilities of today's computers, but the forerunner of the vacuum tube, transistor, magnetic tape, and printed circuits that brought about the information revolution. These two events—the development of radioactive isotopes and the invention of the computer—revolutionized science and provided a new way to explore the most complex structure in existence—the human brain. Today, we can use positron emission tomography to relate our thinking, emotions, and behavior to chemical reactions going on in our brains. We can explore the chemistry of cowardice and courage as well as violence, aggression, love, and hate.

In the past, philosophers, psychiatrists, and psychologists had to rely on soul-searching introspection to try to fathom the workings of the human mind. We can look at both sides now—brain chemistry and behavior. We can measure the sources of energy—glucose and oxygen—within the mind, and the process of neurotransmission, the communication system of the brain. We can see what it takes to live vigorously and enthusiastically. We can begin to learn how to induce chemical changes in the brain—a kind of chemical biofeedback—without taking drugs, either licit or illicit. We can begin to learn how to "turn ourselves on" by observing how our behavior affects our brain chemistry.

A cynical view, accepted by some more than forty years ago and by others even today, is that the peaceful uses of atomic energy are a sop intended by militaristic leaders to convince the public to sustain the development of the military uses of atomic energy. Just after World War II, in 1946, the United Nations passed a resolution to establish the U.N. Atomic Energy Commission "to make proposals for using atomic energy for peaceful purposes, eliminating atomic and other weapons of mass destruction from national armaments, and effectively safeguarding complying states." The commission's stated goal was to reach "a hard-backed, realistic enforceable world agreement that would ensure the outlawing of atomic weapons." Despite the commission's failure to attain that goal, and despite the subsequent nuclear arms race, the world has managed to avoid a nuclear holocaust for nearly half a century. The threat of nuclear war may indeed have had a restraining effect on military operations by the Soviet Union and the United States, but today nearly everyone would agree that the human race is playing with global dynamite. Some would argue that the solution to this ever-volatile threat lies within the human brain rather than in the world of politics and diplomacy.

In his *Principles of Psychology*, William James wrote: "Chemical changes must, of course, accompany mental activity, but little is known of their exact nature." Perception, emotion, thought, memory, attention, will, and consciousness are reflected in the chemistry of the brain. James also wrote that "the relation of a mind to its own brain is of a unique and utterly mysterious sort." That relation can now be explored by positron emission tomography. For the first time, we can examine the patterns and changes in the "recognition" sites on the nerve cells within our brains in relation to our feelings and behavior.

We are all suffering from paranoia, a life-threatening disease that endangers the entire human species. Diagnosis of this disease will require a better understanding of the workings of the human brain, which in turn will enable us to change our modes of thinking. Cure of the disease may depend on whether we can better understand the chemical correlates of our fears and insecurities, our violence and destructiveness, and so declare both sides winners and stop the arms race.

Physics has given us the power to destroy ourselves. Perhaps only biology can save us. The only effective defense against nuclear weapons may lie within the human mind. As William James wrote, "What doctrines students take from their teachers are of little consequence provided they catch from them the living, philosophic attitude of mind, the independent, personal look at all the data of life, and the eagerness to harmonize them."

BIBLIOGRAPHY

The authors hope that the following selection of books presents both sides of the nuclear energy issue. It does not purport to be a comprehensive list, but can provide a starting point for further reading to assess the benefits versus the risks of radiation.

FOREWORD

Seaborg, Glenn T. *Man and Atom*. New York: E. P. Dutton, 1971.
Seaborg, Glenn T. *Nuclear Milestones: A Collection of Speeches by G. T. Seaborg*. San Francisco: W. H. Freeman, 1972.

PROLOGUE: THE POLITICS OF FEAR

The Tin Trial in Malaysia
Bentley, Judith. *The Nuclear Freeze Movement*. New York: F. Watts, 1984.
Caldicott, Helen. *Nuclear Madness*. Brookline, Mass.: Autumn Press, 1978.
Lewis, Richard S. *The Nuclear-Power Rebellion*. New York: Viking Press, 1972.
Price, Jerome. *The Antinuclear Movement*. Boston: Twayne Publishers, 1982.

ONE: THE RADIOACTIVE PLANET EARTH

Uranium
Ardley, Neil. *Atoms and Energy*. New York: Warwick Press, 1982.
Asimov, Isaac. *Inside the Atom*. New York: Abelard-Schuman, 1966.
Eisenbud, Merril. *Environmental Radioactivity: From Natural, Industrial, and Military Sources*. New York: McGraw-Hill, 1963; New York: Academy Press, 1987.
Fradin, Dennis B. *Radiation*. Chicago: Children's Press, 1987.
Freeman, Ira Maximilian. *Light and Radiation*. New York: Holiday House, 1966.
Frisch, Otto Robert. *Working with Atoms*. New York: Basic Books, 1965.
Gesell, T. F., and Lowden, W. M., eds. *The Natural Radiation Environment II*.

Washington, D.C.: Technical Information Center, U.S. Department of Energy, 1975.

Grey, Vivian. *Secret of the Mysterious Rays.* New York: Basic Books, 1966.

Grisanti, Mary Lee. *Rare Earth.* Garden City, N.Y.: Doubleday, 1986.

Haber, Heinz. *Our Friend the Atom.* New York: Simon and Schuster, 1956. Illustrated by the Walt Disney Studio.

Halacy, Daniel Stephen. *Radiation, Magnetism, and Living Things.* New York: Holiday House, 1966.

Hall, Eric J. *Radiation and Life.* Rev. ed. New York: Pergamon Press, 1984.

Jespersen, James, and Fitz-Randolph, Jane. *From Quarks to Quasars: A Tour of the Universe.* New York: Macmillan, 1987.

Jones, G. O.; Rotblat, J.; and Whitrow, G. J. *Atoms and the Universe.* New York: Charles Scribner's Sons, 1956.

Lillie, David W. *Our Radiant World.* Ames: Iowa State University Press, 1986.

Pettigrew, Mark. *Radiation.* New York: Gloucester Press, 1986.

Reinfeld, Fred. *Rays: Visible and Invisible.* New York: Sterling Publishing Co., 1958.

Schwartz, Joe. *Einstein for Beginners.* New York: Pantheon Books, 1979.

Shan, Lawrence Lee, and Margeau, Henry. *Einstein's Space and Van Gough's Sky: Physical Reality and Beyond.* New York: Macmillan, 1982.

Radioactivity

Asimov, Isaac. *How Did We Find Out about Atoms.* New York: Walker and Co., 1976.

Curie, Eve. *Madame Curie: A Biography.* Translated by Vincent Scheean. New York: Doubleday, Doran, and Co., 1938.

del Regato, Juan A. *Radiological Physicists.* New York: American Association of Physicists in Medicine, American Institute of Physics, 1985.

Giroud, Francoise. *Marie Curie: A Life* (une Femme Honorable). Translated by Lydia Davis. New York: Holmes and Meier, 1986.

Holton, Gerald, and Romer, Alfred, eds. *Radiochemistry and the Discovery of Isotopes.* Classics of Science, vol. 6. New York: Dover Publications, 1970.

Lawrence, William Leonard. *Men and Atoms.* New York: Simon and Schuster, 1959.

McKay, Alwyn. *The Making of the Atomic Age.* Oxford: Oxford University Press, 1984.

Romer, Alfred, and Holton, Gerald, eds. *The Discovery of Radioactivity and Transmutation.* New York: Dover Publications, 1964.

See, Carolyn. *Golden Days.* New York: McGraw-Hill, 1987.

Silverberg, Robert. *Men Who Mastered the Atom.* New York: Putnam, 1965.

Trower, W. Peter, ed. *Discovering Alvarez: Selected Works of Luis W. Alvarez with Commentary by His Students and Colleagues.* Chicago: University of Chicago Press, 1987.

Weaver, Jefferson Hane, ed. *The World of Physics: A Small Library of the*

Literature of Physics from Antiquity to the Present. New York: Simon and Schuster, 1987.

The Tracer Principle

Levi, Hilde. *George de Hevesy: Life and Work*. Copenhagen: Rhodos, 1985.

TWO: PLOWSHARES OR SWORDS?

The Birth of the Atomic Bomb

Bernstein, B. J., ed. *The Atomic Bomb*. Boston: Little, Brown, and Co., 1976.

Bernstein, Jeremy. *Hans Bethe: Prophet of Energy*. New York: Basic Books, 1980.

Clark, Ronald William. *The Birth of the Bomb: The Untold Story of Britain's Part in the Weapon that Changed the World*. New York: Horizon, 1960; London: Phoenix House, 1961.

Clark, Ronald William. *The Greatest Power on Earth*. New York: Harper and Row, 1980.

Compton, Arthur Holly. *Atomic Quest*. Oxford: Oxford University Press, 1956.

Davis, Noel Pharr. *Lawrence and Oppenheimer*. New York: Simon and Schuster, 1968.

Fermi, Laura. *Atoms in the Family: My Life with Enrico Fermi*. 1954. Reprint. Albuquerque: University of New Mexico Press, 1988.

"The First Pile." *Bulletin of the Atomic Scientists*, December 1962.

Groves, Leslie R. *Now It Can Be Told*. New York: Harper and Row, 1962; New York: De Capo Press, 1983.

Hawkins, Helen S.; Greb, G. Allen; and Szilard, Gertrude Weiss, eds. *Toward a Livable World: Leo Szilard and the Crusade for Nuclear Arms Control*. Cambridge, Mass.: MIT Press, 1988.

Jungk, Robert. *Brighter Than a Thousand Suns*. New York: Harcourt Brace, 1958.

Lewis, Richard S.; Wilson, Jane; and Rabinowitch, Eugene, eds. *Alamogordo Plus Twenty-Five Years: The Impact of Atomic Energy on Science, Technology, and World Politics*. New York: Viking Press, 1970.

Nathan, Otto, and Norden, Heinz, eds. *Einstein on Peace*. New York: Schocken Books, 1968.

National Academy of Sciences. *Biographical Memoirs*. Vol. 40, *Leo Szilard*. New York: Columbia University Press, 1962.

Nichols, Kenneth David. *The Road to Trinity*. New York: Morrow, 1987.

Oppenheimer, J. Robert. *The Open Mind*. New York: Simon and Schuster, 1955.

Rigden, John S. *Rabi: Scientist and Citizen*. New York: Basic Books, 1988.

Sayen, Jamie. *Einstein in America: The Scientist's Conscience in the Age of Hitler and Hiroshima*. New York: Crown, 1985.

Smith, Martin Cruz. *Stallion's Gate*. New York: Random House, 1986.

Szilard, Gertrude Weiss, and Feld, Bernard T., eds. *The Collected Works of Leo Szilard.* Cambridge, Mass.: MIT Press, 1978.

The Decision

Adams, Ruth, and Cullen, Susan, eds. *The Final Epidemic: Physicians and Scientists on Nuclear War.* Chicago: Educational Foundation for Nuclear Science, 1981.

Caldicott, Helen. *Missile Envy.* New York: Morrow, 1984; New York: Bantam Books, 1986.

Craig, Paul P. *Nuclear Arms Race.* New York: McGraw-Hill, 1985.

Gay, William. *The Nuclear Arms Race.* Chicago: American Library Association, 1987.

Haalan, Carsten M. *Radiation Safety in Shelters.* Written at Oak Ridge National Laboratory under contract with the Federal Emergency Management Agency. Publ. No. CPG 2-6.4, 1983. Available free of charge from FEMA, Box 8181, Washington, D.C., 20024.

Halperin, Morton H. *Nuclear Fallacy: Dispelling the Myth of Nuclear Strategy.* Cambridge, Mass.: Ballinger Publishing Co., 1987.

Hawkes, Nigel. *Nuclear Arms Race.* New York: Gloucester Press, 1986.

Hiroshima and Nagasaki: The Physical, Medical, and Social Effects of the Atomic Bombings. New York: Basic Books, 1981.

Katz, Milton S. *Ban the Bomb: A History of SANE, the Committee for a Sane Nuclear Policy, 1957–1985.* Westport, Conn.: Greenwood Press, 1986.

Loeb, Paul Rogat. *Hope in Hard Times.* Lexington, Mass.: Lexington Books, 1987.

National Academy of Sciences. National Research Council. Commission on Physical Sciences, Mathematics, and Resources. Committee on the Atmospheric Effects of Nuclear Explosions. *The Effects of a Major Nuclear Exchange.* Washington, D.C.: National Academy Press, 1985.

O'Brien, William Vincent, and Langan, John, eds. *The Nuclear Dilemma and the Just War Tradition.* Lexington, Mass.: Lexington Books, 1986.

Pauling, Linus. *No More War!* Westport, Conn.: Greenwood Press, 1975.

Paulson, Dennis. *Voices of Survival in the Nuclear Age.* Santa Barbara, Calif.: Capra Press, 1986.

Russell, Bertrand. *Has Man a Future?* New York: Simon and Schuster, 1961.

Schell, Jonathan. *The Fate of the Earth.* New York: Alfred A. Knopf, 1982.

Scoville, Herbert. *Missile Madness.* Boston: Houghton Mifflin, 1970.

Solomon, Fredric, and Marston, Robert Q. eds. *The Medical Implications of Nuclear War.* Washington, D.C.: National Academy Press, 1986.

Strieber, Whitley, and Kunetka, James. *Warday.* New York: Holt, Rinehart, and Winston, 1984.

Teller, Edward. *The Legacy of Hiroshima.* Garden City, N.Y.: Doubleday, 1962.

Wade, Nicholas. *A World beyond Healing: The Prologue and Aftermath of Nuclear War.* New York: W. W. Norton, 1987.

Zuckerman, Baron Solly. *Star Wars in a Nuclear World*. New York: Vintage Books, 1987.

International Control

Blechman, Barry M. *Preventing Nuclear War: A Realistic Approach*. Bloomington: Indiana University Press in association with the Center for Strategic and International Studies, Georgetown University, Washington, D.C., 1985.

LeBaron, Wayne D. *The Reluctant Survivors: A Family Guide to the Prevention and Treatment of Radiation Sickness*. New York: Bantam Books, 1984.

Leventhal, Paul, and Alexander, Yonah, eds. *Preventing Nuclear Terrorism: The Report and Papers of the International Task Force on Prevention of Nuclear Terrorism*. Lexington, Mass.: Lexington Books, 1987.

The Atomic Energy Act of 1946

Ball, Howard. *Justice Downwind: America's Atomic Testing Program in the 1950's*. New York: Oxford University Press, 1986.

Fuller, John Grant. *The Day We Bombed Utah: America's Most Lethal Secret*. New York: New American Library, 1984.

Hacker, Barton C. *The Dragon's Tail: Radiation Safety in the Manhattan Project, 1942–1946*. Berkeley and Los Angeles: University of California Press, 1987.

Hewlett, Richard G., and Anderson, Oscar Edgar A. *A History of the United States Atomic Energy Commission: The New World, 1939–1946*. University Park: Pennsylvania State University Press, 1962.

Lilienthal, David E. *The Journal of David E. Lilienthal*. Vol. 2, *The Atomic Energy Years, 1945–1950*. New York: Harper and Row, 1964.

Miller, Richard L. *Under the Cloud: The Decades of Nuclear Testing*. New York: Free Press; London: Collier Macmillan, 1986.

Nuse, James D. *Legislative History of the Atomic Energy Act of 1946*. Washington, D.C. U.S. Atomic Energy Commission, 1955.

Titus, A. Costandina. *Bombs in the Backyard: Atomic Testing and American Politics*. Reno: University of Nevada Press, 1950.

Williams, Robert C., and Cantelona, Philip L. *The American Atom: A Documentary History of Nuclear Policies from the Discovery of Fission to the Present, 1939–1984*. Philadelphia: University of Pennsylvania Press, 1984.

THREE: NUCLEAR MEDICINE

The Chemistry of Life

Alazraki, Naomi P., and Mishkin, Fred S. *Fundamentals of Nuclear Medicine*. New York: Society of Nuclear Medicine, 1984.

Greitz, T.; Ingvar, D. H.; and Widen, L., eds. *The Metabolism of the Human Brain Studied with Positron Emission Tomography*. New York: Raven Press, 1985.

Phelps, M. E., and Mazziotta, J. C. "Positron Emission Tomography: Human Brain Function and Biochemistry." *Science* 228(1985):799–809.
Wagner, Henry N., Jr. "Positron Emission Tomography and the Chemistry of Mental Illness." In *Year Book of Nuclear Medicine*, ed. Paul Hoffer et al. Chicago: Year Book Publishers, 1988.

FOUR: LIVING WITH UNCERTAINTY

Radiation and Women

Evans, R. D. "Radium Poisoning: A Review of Present Knowledge." *American Journal of Public Health* 23(1933):1017–1023.
Gossner, W., ed. *The Radiobiology of Radium and Thorotrast*. Baltimore: Urban and Schwarzenberg, 1986.
Loutit, J. F. "Malignancy from Radium." *British Journal of Cancer* 24(1970):195–207.
Martland, H. S. "The Occurrence of Malignancy in Radioactive Persons." *American Journal of Cancer* 15(1931):2455–2516.
Polednak, A. P., Stehney, A. F., and Rowland, R. E. "Mortality among Women First Employed before 1930 in the U.S. Radium-Dial Painting Industry." *American Journal of Epidemiology* 107(1978):179–195.

Three Mile Island and Chernobyl

Adato, Michelle; MacKenzie, James; Pollard, Robert; and Weiss, Ellyn. *Safety Second: The NRC and America's Nuclear Power Plants*. Bloomington: Indiana University Press, 1987.
American Medical Association. *A Guide to the Hospital Management of Injuries Arising from Exposure to or Involving Ionizing Radiation*. OP 335. Chicago: AMA, 1984.
Asimov, Isaac. *How Did We Find Out About Nuclear Power?* New York: Walker and Co., 1976.
Bennett, Donald John. *The Elements of Nuclear Power*. New York: John Wiley and Sons, 1972.
Berger, John J. *Nuclear Power—The Unviable Option: A Critical Look at Our Energy Alternatives*. Palo Alto, Calif.: Ramparts Press, 1976.
Bolt, Bruce A. *Nuclear Explosions and Earthquakes*. San Francisco: W. H. Freeman, 1976.
Camilleri, Joseph A. *The State and Nuclear Power*. Seattle: University of Washington Press, 1984.
Cantelon, Philip L., and Williams, Robert C. *Crisis Contained: The Department of Energy at Three Mile Island*. Carbondale: Southern Illinois University Press, 1982.
Curtis, Richard, and Hogan, Elizabeth. *Perils of the Peaceful Atom: The Myth of Safe Nuclear Power Plants*. Garden City, N.Y.: Doubleday, 1969.
Fuchs, Erich. *What Makes a Nuclear Power Plant Work?* New York: Delacorte Press, 1972.

Haines, Gail Kay. *The Great Nuclear Power Debate*. New York: Dodd, Mead, and Co., 1985.

Hawkes, Nigel. *Chernobyl: The End of the Nuclear Dream*. New York: Vintage Books, 1986.

Hawkes, Nigel. *Nuclear Safety*. New York: Gloucester Press, 1986.

Gale, Robert Peter, and Hauser, Thomas. *Final Warning: The Legacy of Chernobyl*. New York: Warner Books, 1988.

International Atomic Energy Agency. *Summary Report on the Post-Accident Review Meeting on the Chernobyl Accident*. Safety Series No. 75, INSAG-1. Vienna: IAEA, 1986.

Kereiakes, J. G., et al. "The Accident at Chernobyl." *Seminars in Nuclear Medicine* 16(1986):224.

Lebow, Richard Ned. *Nuclear Crisis Management: A Dangerous Illusion*. Ithaca, N.Y.: Cornell University Press, 1987.

Marples, David R. *Chernobyl and Nuclear Power in the USSR*. New York: St. Martin's Press in association with the Canadian Institute of Ukrainian Studies, University of Alberta, 1986.

Medvedev, Zhores A. *Nuclear Disaster in the Urals*. Translated by George Saunders. New York: W. W. Norton, 1979.

Pohl, Frederik. *Chernobyl*. New York: Bantam Books, 1987.

President's Commission on the Accident at Three Mile Island. *Reports of the Public Health and Safety Task Force on Public Health and Safety Summary, Health Physics and Dosimetry, Radiation Health Effects, Behavioral Effects, Public Health and Epidemiology*. Washington, D.C.: Government Printing Office, 1979.

Sills, David L.; Wolf, C. P.; and Shelanski, Vivien B. *Accident at Three Mile Island: The Human Dimensions*. Boulder, Colo.: Westview Press, 1982.

Tomain, Joseph P. *Nuclear Power Transformation*. Bloomington: Indiana University Press, 1987.

U.S. Congress. House. Committee on Science and Technology. Subcommittee on Energy Research and Production. *Nuclear Power Plant Safety after Three Mile Island*. 96th Cong., 2nd sess., 1980.

Webster, Edward W. "Chernobyl Predictions and the Chinese Contribution." *Journal of Nuclear Medicine* 28(1987):423–425.

Nuclear Waste Disposal: Not in My Backyard

Barlett, Donald L., and Steele, James B. *Forevermore: Nuclear Waste in America*. New York: W. W. Norton, 1985; pbk. ed., 1986.

Murray, Raymond L. *Understanding Radioactive Waste*. 2nd ed. Columbus, Ohio: Battelle Press, 1983.

Radon Becomes a Household Word

Cohen, Bernard. *Radon: A Homeowner's Guide to Detection and Control*. Consumer Reports Books. Mount Vernon, N.Y.: Consumers Union, 1987.

Ginevan, M. E., and Mills, W. A. "Assessing the Risks of Radon Exposure: The Influence of Cigarette Smoking." *Health Physician* 51(1986):163–174.

National Academy of Sciences. National Research Council. Committee on the Biological Effects of Ionizing Radiations. *Health Risks of Radon and Other Internally Deposited Alpha-Emitters* (BEIR IV Report). Washington, D.C.: National Academy Press, 1988.

Thomas, D. C., McNeill, K. G., and Doutherty, C. "Estimates of Lifetime Lung Cancer Risks Resulting from Radon Progeny Exposures." *Health Physician* 49(1985):825–846.

U.S. Environmental Protection Agency. *A Citizen's Guide to Radon: What It Is and What to Do*. Washington, D.C.: EPA, 1986.

Wadden, Richard A., and Scheff, Peter A. *Indoor Air Pollution: Characterization, Prediction, and Control*. New York: John Wiley and Sons, 1983.

Gamma Rays for Gourmets

Elias, P. S., and Cohen, A. J., eds. *Recent Advances in Food Irradiation*. Amsterdam: Elsevier, 1983.

Urbain, Walter M. *Food Irradiation*. Orlando, Fla.: Academic Press, 1986.

Webb, Tony; Lang, Tim; and Tucker, Kathleen. *Food Irradiation: Who Wants It?* Rochester, Vt.: Thorsons Publishers, 1987; distributed by Harper and Row.

FIVE: THE SEARCH FOR TRUTH

Fighting Ignorance and Fear

Lichter, S. Robert; Rothman, Stanley; Rycroft, Robert W.; and Lichter, Linda S. *Nuclear News*. Washington, D.C.: Center for Media and Public Affairs, 1986.

Loeb, Paul Rogat. *Nuclear Culture: Living and Working in the World's Largest Atomic Complex*. Philadelphia: New Society Publishers, 1986.

The Scientific Method

Barnes, Barry. *About Science*. Oxford and New York: Basil Blackwell Ltd., 1985.

Efron, Edith. *The Apocalyptics: How Environmental Politics Controls What We Know about Cancer*. New York: Simon and Schuster, 1984.

Smith, Alan G. R. *Science and Society in the Sixteenth and Seventeenth Centuries*. London: Thames and Hudson, Ltd.; New York: Harcourt Brace Jovanovich, 1972.

How to Choose

Douglas, Mary Tew, and Wildavsky, Aaron. *Risk and Culture*. Berkeley and Los Angeles: University of California Press, 1983.

Viscusi, W. Kip. *Risk by Choice: Regulating Health and Safety in the Workplace*. Cambridge, Mass.: Harvard University Press, 1983.

Risk Perception and Risk Assessment

Boice, J. D., Jr., and Fraumeni, J. F., Jr., eds. *Radiation Carcinogenesis: Epidemiology and Biological Significance*. New York: Raven Press, 1984.

Brill, Bertrand A., ed. *Low-Level Radiation Effects: A Fact Book*. New York: Society of Nuclear Medicine, 1982, 1985.

Cohen, Bernard Leonard. *Nuclear Science and Society*. Garden City, N.Y.: Anchor Press, 1974.

Dowling, David. *Fictions of Nuclear Disaster*. Iowa City: University of Iowa Press, 1987.

Fabrikant, Jacob I. *Radiobiology*. Chicago: Year Book Medical Publishers, 1972.

Freeman, Leslie J. *Nuclear Witnesses: Insiders Speak Out*. New York: W. W. Norton, 1981.

Glendinning, Chellis. *Waking Up in the Nuclear Age: The Book of Nuclear Therapy*. New York: Beech Tree Books, 1987.

Gofman, John William. *Radiation and Human Health*. New York: Pantheon Books, 1983.

GPU Nuclear Corporation. *Radiation and Health Effects: A Report on the TMI-2 Accident and Related Health Studies*. Middleton, Pa.: GPU Nuclear Corp., 1986.

Hayes, Dennis. *Rays of Hope*. New York: W. W. Norton, 1977.

Hyde, Margaret O. *Atoms Today and Tomorrow*. New York: McGraw-Hill, 1970.

International Commission on Radiological Protection. *Limits on Intake of Radionuclides by Workers*. ICRP Publication No. 30. Oxford: Pergamon Press, 1979.

Jones, Claire. *Pollution: The Dangerous Atom*. Minneapolis: Lerner Publications Co., 1972.

La Farge, Phyllis. *The Strangelove Legacy: Children, Parents, and Teachers in the Nuclear Age*. New York: Harper and Row, 1987.

Lifton, Robert Jay. *"The Future of Immortality" and Other Essays for a Nuclear Age*. New York: Basic Books, 1987.

Mettler, F. A., and Moseley, F. D. *Medical Effects of Ionizing Radiation*. Orlando, Fla.: Grune and Stratton, 1985.

Moche, Dinah L. *Radiation, Benefits/Dangers*. New York: Watts, 1979.

Morgan, Karl Ziegler. *Principles of Radiation Protection*. New York: John Wiley and Sons, 1967.

National Academy of Sciences. National Research Council. Committee on the Biological Effects of Ionizing Radiations. *The Effects on Populations of Exposure to Low Levels of Ionizing Radiation* (BEIR III Report). Washington, D.C.: National Academy Press, 1980.

National Council on Radiation Protection and Measurements. *Ionizing Radiation Exposure of the Population of the United States*. NCRP Report No. 93. Bethesda, Md.: NCRP, 1987.

National Council on Radiation Protection and Measurements. *Recommenda-*

tions on Limits for Exposure to Ionizing Radiation. NCRP Report No. 91. Bethesda, Md.: NCRP, 1987.

Ott, John Nash. *Light, Radiation, and You.* Old Greenwich, Conn.: Devin Adair Co., 1982.

Panati, Charles. *The Silent Intruder.* Boston: Houghton Mifflin, 1981.

Polking, Kirk. *Let's Go to an Atomic Energy Town.* New York: G. P. Putnam's, 1968.

Radiation Effects Research Foundation. *U.S.-Japan Joint Reassessment of Atomic Bomb Radiation Dosimetry in Hiroshima and Nagasaki.* Final Report. Edited by W. C. Roesch. Hiroshima: RERF, 1987.

Shannon, Sara. *Diet for the Atomic Age: How to Protect Yourself from Low-Level Radiation.* Garden City, N.Y.: Avery Publishing Group, 1987.

U.N. Scientific Committee on the Effects of Atomic Radiation. *Sources and Effects of Ionizing Radiation.* UNSCEAR Report E.77.IX.1. New York: United Nations, 1977.

Woodbury, David Oakes. *The New World of the Atom.* New York: Dodd, Mead, and Co., 1965.

ORGANIZATIONS CONCERNED WITH RADIATION ISSUES

American Council on Science and Health, 47 Maple Street, Summit, N.J. 07901

American Nuclear Society, 555 North Kensington Avenue, La Grange Park, Ill. 60525

Center for Risk Management Resources for the Future, 1616 P Street, Washington, D.C. 20036

Committee on Interagency Radiation Research and Policy Coordination (CIRRPC), 1019 Nineteenth Street N.W., Suite 700, Washington, D.C. 20036

Health Physics Society, 8000 Westpark Drive, Suite 400, McLean, Va. 22102

International Atomic Energy Agency (IAEA), Vienna International Center, Wagramerstrasse 5, P.O. Box 100, A-1400 Vienna, Austria

National Council on Radiation Protection and Measurements (NCRP), 7910 Woodmont Avenue, Bethesda, Md. 20814

The Society of Nuclear Medicine (SNM), Committee on Biologic Effects of Radiation, 136 Madison Avenue, New York, N.Y. 10016

Union of Concerned Scientists, 26 Church Street, Cambridge, Mass. 02238

United Nations Scientific Committee on the Effects of Atomic Radiation (UNSCEAR), Vienna International Center, Wagramerstrasse 5, P.O. Box 500, A-1400 Vienna, Austria

U.S. Council for Energy Awareness, 1776 "Eye" Street, N.W., Suite 400, Washington, D.C. 20006-2495

U.S. Department of Energy (DOE), Office of Public Affairs, Washington, D.C. 20585

U.S. Environmental Protection Agency (EPA), Office of Radiation Programs, 401 M Street S.W., Mail Code ANR-458, Washington, D.C. 20460
U.S. Environmental Protection Agency (EPA), Radon Action Program, 401 M Street S.W., Mail Code ANR-460, Washington, D.C. 20460
U.S. Nuclear Regulatory Commission (NRC), Washington, D.C. 20555

INDEX

Henry N. Wagner, Jr., M.D., is Director of the Divisions of Nuclear Medicine and Radiation Health Sciences and professor of medicine, radiology, and environmental health sciences at the Johns Hopkins University School of Medicine. Linda E. Ketchum is senior medical editor and writer at ProClinica, Inc., in New York.

Designed by Martha Farlow

Text composed by Action Comp, Inc., in Paladium and display lines composed by Charles Street Graphics in Syntax Bold

Printed by R. R. Donnelley & Sons Company on 55-lb. Cream White Sebago and bound in Holliston Aqualite